Something More Than Hope

"Diana and Kelly Lindsay have written a remarkable account of Diana's exceptional recovery from stage 4 lung cancer. They faced daunting odds with fierce intentionality and a wise integration of conventional and integrative therapies. Above all, they understand the healing power of love. A beautiful story, well told."

— Michael Lerner, President and Founder, Commonweal

"Diana and Kelly's moving journeys in the face of cancer affirm that miracles are made — not with blueprints or instruction manuals, but with courage, intuition, intelligence and abiding love. The honesty, humor and insights embedded in each chapter are unique to them as patient and caretaker, wife and husband, yet universal in their depiction of the human heart as it opens and closes and opens again to the onslaught of life in all its rawness and beauty. For those with a life-threatening illness and their loved ones, this book is like a dear friend at your side, reminding you that you are not alone, whatever your path may be."

— Elise Miller, MEd
Director, Collaborative on Health and the Environment

"This book is profoundly engaging and provides an example of transformational learning at its best. It opens up new worlds of possibility for the healing of body, mind and soul, and in that sense it is truly revolutionary."

— Susanne M. Fest, Ed.d.,
Social Science Concentration Chair,
Individualized Master of Arts,
Antioch University Midwest

"Diana and Kelly's companion books bring deep and astonishing new ways of thinking. The humor and the bluntness, the compassion and the clarity, the insights and the inspiration are all great guides for us. Both books have breathtaking images that catapult us into sensation, experience, and empathy and uplift us with their light and lightness."

—Tandy Beal, Artistic Director, Tandy Beal and Company, and director of shows for Moscow Circus, Nightmare Before Christmas, Carl Sagan, and many more

"The clinical insights are profound and continually inspiring. The uncharted inner journey had me hanging on every page."

— Victoria Locke, breast cancer survivor

"We read the book to each other and shared all the emotional ups and downs, visions and hopes that your story triggered in our minds. Both Diana and Kelly were able to express the fears, regrets, and questions that we were afraid to express to ourselves and to each other. Thank you so much for the hope you have given us! You don't know how your words have opened our hearts to face this new life with determination and a clear goal."

— Sara Giswold, caregiver of spouse newly diagnosed with stage 4 ductal carcinoma

Something More Than Hope

*Surviving despite the odds,
thriving because of them*

Diana Lindsay

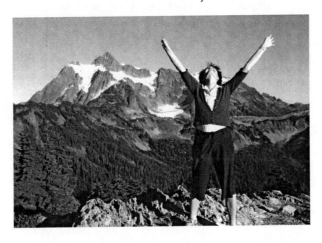

Inroads Press

Inroads Press
P.O. Box 1308
534 Camano Avenue
Langley, WA 98260
inroadspress.com

The authors are grateful for use of the following copyrighted material:

The photographs are by permission of Diana & Kelly Lindsay with the following exceptions:

Tandy Beal & Company for photographs from the production of *HereAfterHere*. Photographs by Chunyi McIver.

Royalty-free stock images by Sebastian Kaulitzki (*dreamstime.com*).

Creative Commons photographs by Shane Porter.

Image reprinted from *The American Journal of Pathology,* vol. 163, Carol A. de la Motte, "Mononuclear Leukocytes Bing to Specific Hyaluronan Structures on Colon Mucosal Smooth Muscle Cells Treated with Polyinosinic Acid", page 121, copyright 2003, with permission from Elsevier.

Images reprinted from *Cell biology of the Extracellular Matrix,* ed. Elizabeth D. Hay, (NY: Plenum Press, 1991). With kind permission from Springer Science and Business Media.

Book design by Morgan Bondelid

Printed in the United States of America

ISBN 978-0-9912427-0-2

For our grandchildren

Even after all this time,
the sun never says to the earth,
"You owe me."
Look what happens with a love like that.
It lights the whole sky.

—Hafiz

Contents

Authors' Foreword

Sixteen minutes is the average lead time we get from a tornado warning. Just sixteen minutes to race to your children or grandchildren, grab them under your arm, and run to the nearest shelter. There isn't, however, an average recovery time. How long before we emerge from the shelter, stand on the ruin of a former home, and rebuild a life is up to us. It takes about four seconds to hear the words "You have cancer," "I want a divorce," or "I'm sorry for your loss." The rubble at your feet may not be shattered glass and splintered wood, but the devastation feels comparable.

The brain has difficulty handling these moments of utter vulnerability. Our common understandings of the world and habitual responses rip away like roof shingles in a 200 mile-per-hour wind. We might sob with anguish or stare blankly, but in that moment we are usually incapable of taking in anything else. And yet, most of us recover. Brain circuits reboot and begin processing again. We look around, sense a direction, and take a step forward. We are hardwired for resilience.

When we were told Diana had a terminal illness, at first we didn't believe there could be any way we could survive the blow. When Diana decided to pick up and start moving, our expectations were minimal. We had no way of knowing that the trek would revitalize our marriage, transform how we live and love, and deeply connect us to healing sources within us and in the world at large. We didn't yet have the imagination to conceive of a Love-In, a Gratitude Tour, a Cuddle Shuttle, or Skyping Diana's cells—much less acknowledge them as messengers of healing.

We didn't have a clue that we would benefit along the way from Western medicine's latest advances in destroying cancer cells and Eastern energy medicine's guidance on strengthening our healthy cells. It was precisely the extreme narrowing of Diana's treatment options that forced us to expand our thinking enough to discover how to make our own medicine. It was only after losing the comfort of any familiar path that she discovered her body could guide her through the unknown.

If you've begun to read at this point, from here to the middle of the book you'll find Diana's story. It's about what happens when life both demands—and offers—*Something More Than Hope.* Starting from the opposite end of the book you'll find Kelly's perspective on the same story, about giving up—and getting back—*Something More Than Everything* in his role as Diana's primary caregiver. If you find yourself facing illness, catastrophe, or despair, we hope our story will ease your way as you find your own.

This book is not only about cancer. There are many moments in life when we are thrust into a bear pit that seems to have no way out but through the bear. It is not even about coming to a happy ending. It's about the hope and creativity, love and joy, awe and gratitude that come from drinking in every moment we're alive—no matter how many days we have left.

CHAPTER ONE

When Medicine Comes Up Short

January–May, 2006

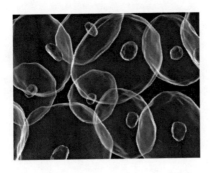

This is a mystery novel without a dead body. It was just a simple breath that alerted the detectives. Looking back on it, clues were scattered everywhere. Still, I was right there, and I missed them all.

Doctors are trained with the mantra, "If you hear hoofbeats in Texas, think horses, not zebras." But I'm trained as a marketing consultant, and I'm far too busy to listen to my body, or think much about my health. Okay, I can't walk uphill as quickly as my client can, but we're in mile-high Mexico City, and she's a recreational bicycle racer. My shoulder hurts, but that's what comes of slinging luggage into overhead compartments on frequent business trips. And the reason I can't shake this cough is probably a sinus infection. But when I'm unable to blow out the candles on my birthday cake, no easy explanation comes to mind; I just laugh, embarrassed.

The embarrassment grows the following week, when I'm in the middle of a brainstorming meeting with another client. I'm busy filling the white board with marketing strategies for his Global 100 company when my coughing gets so bad I have to leave the room. My client follows me out into the corridor and tactfully suggests I see a doctor. I owe him a lot.

I schedule an appointment the next week with an Ear, Nose, and Throat specialist who confirms that my sinuses look like the underground sewer system of an ancient city, and schedules me for surgery. During the routine pre-op checkup, I tell my primary care provider, Cathy Robinson, the story about the birthday cake. She responds by quietly handing me a blow-into-this lung function test. I fail it.

"I'm sorry, Diana, but I'm not buying sinus infection for the cough," she says, as she walks me across the street to get an X-ray. Hours later, she asks me to come back for a CT scan "to check for pneumonia." It's only when her office nurse asks me to prep for an abdominal CT as well that I start worrying that they're checking for something more than pneumonia. So later that day my husband, Kelly, and I are quiet as we sit on our green couch waiting for Cathy's call with the results.

At 4:00 the phone rings.

"Diana, you have lung cancer."

"Are you kidding?" I ask her.

Seriously. I said that.

Of course she isn't kidding. Doctors don't kid about this kind of thing. And Cathy is my friend. I ask her what stage of cancer we're looking at, thinking this will determine whether my next few months will just include surgery or the full complement of surgery, chemotherapy, and radiation that my friends have had to endure with later-stage cancer.

"I can't tell you the stage from this CT," she answers. "But it's at least two and maybe three. The tumor is large, Diana, and it might have penetrated your shoulder."

I turn to Kelly in shock. We have been here once before, when I was diagnosed with colon cancer at an early stage. Both then and now he is the first to register his emotions; my psychological barricades go up before the phone call is even over. Instead of allowing myself to consider that the cancer may have spread, I think of it only as worse-than-before. For a few moments Kelly and I cling to each other on the couch, and then I shift into action mode. We have to tell the kids. We have to pack. We have to leave the apartment.

This apartment is our temporary home. When my sister-in-law, Susan, told me that her husband, Kel's brother, Tom, had left his job and wanted to start a new business, Kelly and I had suggested that they come and stay in our house during the transition. This way they could try out life in the Northwest, save some money, and we could live in the apartment above our office that doubled as a conference room. Everyone loved the idea, so they moved into our home on Whidbey Island in Washington State's Puget Sound, and we moved 15 minutes away to our office in the little town of Langley.

The apartment has a stunning view of the Cascade Mountains and the waters of Saratoga Passage, and we have loved our time in it. But we can't stay here now. I can't go through what I imagine chemo to be like while I'm living right above the office. I refuse to be in the overhead bathroom puking while our staff talks to clients about tools for inter-departmental collaboration. Nor can we go home. Tom and Susan have decided to stay on Whidbey and have already bought a new house—right next door to ours—but they can't move in for another three months.

So Kel and I put a few necessities in a suitcase: sweaters, pants, socks, and underwear. Everything else we own instantly falls into the category of Things We Don't Need. My identity as president of a company now falls into the category of Things That Don't Matter. What matters is family, so we get in the car to drive to Seattle to see our daughter, Camilla, and our son-in-law, Isaac. We hope we'll know what to say when we get there.

⊙ ⊙ ⊙

It's not unusual for us to call and let Camilla and Isaac know that we're coming over. Nine months earlier Camilla gave birth to our first grandchild, Thea. We're crazy in love with her, so we try to visit them whenever we can. Three adults typically sit in the living room working on their laptops while the fourth plays with Thea, in rotating 30-minute shifts. If I have to go to a meeting I return there at night, sleeping with Kelly in the attic room. So Camilla and Isaac suspect nothing out of the ordinary when we walk in the door. They stand in the kitchen with dishtowels in their hands.

How do you tell your own children that your life is at risk? We do it as quickly as possible. Kel blurts out, "Well, Mom went to see Cathy for her cough. Got an X-ray, then a CT scan. And it turns out Mom has lung cancer."

After a moment of disbelief, Camilla and Isaac hug us and offer to let us stay with them while I go through treatment. It's an open-ended, open-hearted invitation, an act of love unburdened by information. We all assume that afterwards life will resume as it was before, but we're a long way from knowing anything. We don't even know what we should be feeling, so we just sit. Together.

⊙⊙⊙

Why am I not completely freaking out? Because, as I mentioned, I've been here before. Thirteen years earlier, in 1993, I successfully fought rectal cancer. Now, during these first days of shock, I stay focused by believing life will repeat itself.

So what do I already know?

1. *I know the importance of perseverance and speed in getting the right diagnosis.* Patients often struggle to get appointments to get diagnosed, and to my mind this just isn't acceptable. Cathy, our doctor, has already been quick to get me the chest X-ray, CT scan, and ultrasound, to see if the cancer has spread to the fluid around my heart. We're going with a local surgeon for the biopsy because he can do it right away. I believe it's critical to work the system urgently, and not to let my own fear slow things down.
2. *I know to find the best possible doctor.* Research shows that where a cancer patient is treated first makes the most

difference in survival.[1] During my bout with rectal cancer the first surgeon I met said he had no idea how he would operate on a rectal tumor so close to my sphincter. I told him I knew and called Ward Trueblood, the gifted chief of surgery at El Camino Hospital in Mountain View, California. My fifteen years of survival without a colostomy are testimony to the importance of that decision. This time I already know I need the biggest guns in western medicine so I want to get into the Seattle Cancer Care Alliance: a collaboration of the Fred Hutchinson Research Institute, the University of Washington Medicine, and Seattle Children's Hospital, it is one of the premier cancer centers in the world.

3. *I know that I get clear and calm the day after diagnosis. I can make difficult medical decisions.* The shock of the diagnosis cleans my mind's house; the non-essential falls away and I can recognize what is most important.

4. *I know how essential the support of family and friends is to my recovery.* We were at a high school football game when I told my friends about the rectal cancer. One friend immediately volunteered to manage a pre-Internet phone tree. I dubbed the people on that list my "spiritual army," and I counted myself fortunate to have so many who cared. It's time to recruit again.

5. *I know that preparation before surgery can positively impact the speed of my recovery.* In 1993 I got the pathology report on a Thursday and was immediately scheduled for surgery the following Tuesday. We flew down to the Bay Area and met with the surgeon Monday morning. The tumor in my rectum was so close to my vagina that he warned me that he might have to take everything out. He also warned

me that I faced the possibility of a permanent colostomy. The day before surgery my friend April asked me if she could try an ancient Japanese healing art called Jin Shin Jyutsu that aims to harmonize life energy. I didn't have a clue what she was doing, or why, but I was grateful for her loving touch. In the meditative quiet an image came to me of a sword protecting my vagina and two lions protecting either side of my rectum. For reasons I couldn't explain, I believed these images were portents, and they lessened my fears. As I was wheeled in for surgery I was calm, and my body was ready. It turned out my vagina was unharmed, my colon could be resected, and I recovered quickly after one setback that required a temporary colostomy.

6. *I know I can deal with the tough stuff.* I can tell my children I have cancer. I can plan for my care, and I have strategies for working through pain. I can get up and walk around the nurse's station when told to do so. I can handle uncertainty. I turned that six months with a temporary colostomy into a semi-scientific experiment. So bring it on: I can handle this one, too.

7. *I know that laughter and energy work helped me with both pain and recovery.* My sense of humor remained intact throughout my experience with cancer that year. Although at first I thought Jin Shin Jyutsu was a little out there, I had my first pain-free hour post-surgery after April used her healing touch.

8. *I know that I will cry when it feels safe to—and not before.* For a month after diagnosis, I held my emotions in check. It was only after I saw my nurse flinch when she first changed my colostomy bag that I let tears flow. The doctor came in and chewed me out. "After two surgeries and all

you've been through, why are you crying now?" "Because I can," I replied. Because the situation wasn't life-threatening any more.

9. *I know I can have conversations with my body.* This knowledge might be most important of all, but more on that later.

10. *I know that I have faced cancer before, and survived.*

Circling the Wagons

It seems inconceivable that Kelly and I could spend seventeen years building up a business and step away from it in less than seventeen hours.

When I had cancer the first time, working through it was never in question. I was going to survive and at 41 our family needed our fledgling company to survive as well. We had no savings and Camilla was just two years away from college. Kelly sat in the hospital room chair awkwardly balancing a heavy 1990s laptop as I dictated emails even as I was punching the patient-controlled analgesic pump for pain relief after surgery.

But this time is different. Compared to losing my life, losing my livelihood is not my biggest concern. At some level, I'm aware that for the last year and for the first time, we have set aside money in a Rainy Day Fund—probably an early warning signal from my body. It's enough to last through a first round of chemotherapy and if it runs out, we are now old enough to have retirement funds we can dip into. We don't talk about the possibility that I won't need them. Retirement? Money? Future? I'm still too stunned for any of these to really register. All I hear is a loud cry from my intuition: I can't continue to fill my life with stress if I'm trying to empty it of cancer. And if I can't get better, then I want to spend every instant I have remaining with those I love.

But I'm still responsible for 15 families' livelihoods—a big enough challenge when I was healthy. I don't want my lack of focus to jeopardize our employees' mortgages so Kelly calls our strategic business partner, Nancy, and receives an immediate reply from her saying, in her typically compassionate way, that she is there for me and for the company and will help take over the day-to-day operations if I want her to. The next morning we meet with our staff at Lindsay Communications. It's the first time I've broken down in front of anyone but Kel. We have all come so far together and now I'm going on leave, whether for a short time or forever none of us knows. As I meet with each person individually they volunteer suggestions for how the company can adjust to no longer having me in the lead.

Mine is not the first tragedy the company has faced this year. Our operations manager lost her husband in a helicopter crash in October. Two weeks later our office manager lost her husband to mesothelioma. It seems to me that our little company is getting far more than its fair share of rotten luck, and I hope my illness isn't the fatal blow—but I have to leave that in other people's hands. I close my eyes as I close the front door behind me and drive off to get a biopsy.

By day I am on a tear. By night doubts tear through me. Do I have enough fight in me to take on this cancer? In the overall scheme of things, does it matter if I gain a few more months—or dare I say years? Is it really worth the effort—and expense—to keep me alive? We all die someday, why not today?

I was 39 when I had cancer the first time. Then the answers to those questions were absolutely clear. No way was I going to saddle my children with the trauma of their mother dying when they were young. But this time Camilla and our son Eric are grown and married. They love me, but I know they could survive my death with the same strength and creativity they have already brought to the rest of their lives. Kelly would be devastated, but I figure this is the price of marriage; one of us has to go first, and I am selfish enough to prefer that it be me.

So tonight, lying in the dark, it is Thea, our first grandchild, who galvanizes my will to live. I ache to sing and dance with her as she grows up. I want her to be old enough to remember how deeply I love her. Thea is also the saving grace for everyone else in our family as we watch her laugh, unaware of any reason why she shouldn't. Not only does she keep Camilla and Isaac preoccupied, but Kelly sleeps with her on his chest, and Tom and Susan's sons, John and Jake, cope by rolling on the floor with her. When I need to escape the crowd to grieve in silence, I take Thea with me for a walk, singing to her until my breath gives out. Holding her in the sling on my chest is a stolen moment of bliss that whispers to me, "Live. Why not?"

My family has gathered. Do you know that look on the faces of your loved ones when they want to help you but don't know how? Maybe they can find the words to say they love you and maybe they can't, but in either case it's a short conversation. And then what? We can hug each other, but unless you're married to the other person, or they're under the age of five, this starts to get uncomfortable pretty quickly. Take a walk together? Sure, but I'm coughing incessantly so a walk doesn't last very long. Cook? Who's supposed to do the cooking? Now that I'm newly designated as sick, do I sit on the couch as if I'm unable to do what I did last week? Should I just pretend this isn't happening? Or stay in bed all day?

And then my sister-in-law Susan gets an email from April, the Jin Shin Jyutsu practitioner, who recommends that everyone hold my fingers and toes to build up my energy. In her book, *My Stroke of Insight,* Jill Bolte Taylor says that recognizing energy is the right brain's job. This is good, because the analytical part of my left brain is fighting the message. "Hold my fingers and toes and cure stage 4 cancer? Give me a break," is my first thought before I break into laughter. Laughter is its own medicine though, and we're all willing to give April's suggestion a try, just like we would any other parlor game. And why not? We have nothing better to do.

Carl Jung said, "There are things in the psyche which I do not produce, but which produce themselves and have their own life." I know what he's talking about. After two surgeries in rapid succession for rectal cancer in 1993, my catheter had been in for four weeks. Two attempts to remove it had already failed. It was extremely painful. One night as I sank into pre-sleep twilight, I sensed a woman at the foot of my bed, curled in a fetal position.

'You are my bladder,' I observed, without a moment's hesitation.

'Yes,' she said.

'Damn,' I thought, 'you look as miserable as I do.' As a mother, I knew exactly what to do with someone in pain: I cradled her, hugging her as we rocked together. 'I can't take this any more,' Bladder Woman said. 'I'm exhausted, please let me sleep.'

'I can see how tired you are. I'm tired too. Can we make a deal? We'll sleep tonight, but in the morning, we need to be done with this catheter nonsense. In the morning the catheter has to go.'

'Deal.'

In the morning, after so many days and failed attempts, the catheter came out uneventfully, and I peed. I had trusted dreams and images before, but I'd never had a two-way conversation with my body, so I relegated this to the dustbin of experiences too weird to reconcile with logic, promptly forgetting all about it. But life-threatening cancer has sharpened my mind. I remember. After the biopsy on my lung, locked in insomnia, too scared to stay awake, too frightened to go to sleep, an image of Lung Woman spontaneously arises.

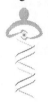

She is a woman my age lying on the tarmac in the dark, pinned underneath a giant boulder. I hurry over and try repeatedly to lift the boulder off her chest, but it's much too heavy. So I crawl down and fit my body next to hers. I hold her and tell her I will wait with her until the medics arrive.

I vaguely hear a helicopter in the distance. As I continue to hold the trapped Lung Woman, twelve, goddess-like figures emerge from my body and form a protective circle around us.

'We are the healthy organs in your body,' they say. 'We will wait with you.'

The next morning I send out an email asking my friends on Whidbey to come wait with me as well. I hope maybe twelve will come.

The Love-In

To: My friends whose email addresses I have
From: Diana
Date: April 27, 2006
Subject: The Great South Whidbey Love In

Hi my loved ones,

Whenever any of you gets sick with cancer I want to give you a big hug—but worry about tiring you. I want to know how you're doing—but worry about bugging the family. I want to help—but there's never much to do. I end up feeling guilty that I was so little help and you had such a struggle.

So I'd like to spare you all that. I want to see you all but have little time before starting chemo. And since I will miss the party season on Whidbey, I invite you to come to the Great Whidbey Love-In at our home on Sunday from 5–8. Bring food, a blanket or a chair, and hope the weather's good.

And since I know you pretend you've attended '60s love-ins and never did, here are the rules:

1. Hug me, hug my family, and hug all my friends. That should be plenty for everyone.
2. Don't ask anyone or talk about medical stuff. See below for the update, and there won't be any more news until my appointment Monday at the Seattle Cancer Care Alliance.
3. Don't bother conjecturing about where this came from or where it will go. Love-ins are all about the present.
4. Enjoy laughing, singing, and dancing with friends. Or act mature and just engage in scintillating conversation while holding a beer.
5. Hot sex is encouraged, but remember to tie a sock on the door of the room or the branch of the bush so no one will interrupt, because at our age the sight would just be too disturbing.

I love you all, and feel free to extend the invitation to anyone who cares about our family.

Diana

P.S. The Medical Stuff

I have been diagnosed with lung cancer. They do not yet know whether they've found the primary site. It is not from my colon cancer of years ago, and CTs don't show it in my abdomen or my brain. It appears to be advanced and chemo looks like the treatment, although we will know more on Monday. I have never had a drag on a cigarette so I fall into a small class of women that seems to be growing.

They come pouring down the hill in twos and threes, bearing platters of food, picnic tables, loudspeakers, guitars, and a washtub bass. I had needed to hug my friends and 125 of them have answered the call. Some may have wondered if they were coming to a So-You're-Going-To-Die advance wake, but wives cajoled husbands into coming, and friends encouraged other friends. Enough have dressed up in remnants of their '60s youth to lighten moments in the serpentine reception line of people waiting to hug me. And in the timeless moment of each embrace, everything really is okay.

What began as a short, spontaneous event, quickly transforms into ritual. Kel's sister, Nancy, brings pink beads for everyone to make bracelets that they will wear for me. A local band, the Rural Characters, starts to sing *I've Got a Never-ending Love for You* and we sing along, husbands holding wives, parents holding children. A friend borrows a guitar and belts out *I am Woman*. I start a long snake line and, for the first time in my life, most people join in. It's hard to say no to a dying woman.

The next morning we find forty socks tied to bushes, door-knobs, and the barbecue (I have to believe most of these were symbolic), and I marvel at the lesson of the Love-In. At 5:00 when it began, I had worried that I would be too sick to stand for the three hours it was scheduled to last. At 11:00 p.m., when it actually ended, I felt exhilarated and deeply joyful.

I felt better.

What had happened in between? There had been no *medical* intervention but there had been a *healing* intervention. We had laughed, danced and sung. We were encircled in a 100-friend hug. I had been radiantly happy in every fiber of my body.

It's not that I thought I deserved to have so many caring friends and family come to my side on a Sunday afternoon. In fact, I had spent much of my life in frenetic service to others in order to overcome a fundamental sense of unworthiness. I had believed that asking for help and taking care of myself were somehow selfish. But my friends had just given me a gift of love with no strings attached; I didn't need to earn it or be worthy of it, just to accept it. Something deep inside me felt freed.

The Love-In reminds me of the things that make *me* feel better, so now I have the first inklings of *my* healing plan. More importantly, I am beginning to believe I am worth the effort of carrying it out.

Stuffing the Doctor's Office

The next day at the Seattle Cancer Care Alliance I'm given a green card, on which is printed my name, my patient ID, my date of birth, my age at admittance, and the fact that I am female. I'm trading my corporate plastic for a patient card, but like the American Express card I'm leaving behind, this membership has its privileges.

I have a patient coordinator who will schedule all my blood tests, CT and MRI scans, and doctor visits as closely to each other as possible; my time, not the doctor's, takes priority. I have a nurse coordinator who will get in touch with my doctor and handle any medical or prescription issues. I have a pharmacy open seven days a week that handles any refill issues directly with my physician. I have been given the right to be treated with respect, to get into my appointments within 15 minutes of their scheduled time, and to have all my online medical records available to anyone within the University of Washington medical system to whom I have allowed access. I sit in waiting rooms that are as lovely as they are clean. Most importantly, I have access to leading-edge medical care and clinical trials linked to the Fred Hutchinson Cancer Research Center.

There is one more perk. On this one embossed card I am, and will always be, 54 years old.

Eight of us cram into the examining room: Kelly and I; Camilla, Isaac, and baby Thea; Isaac's brother, Seth, his wife, Molly, and their baby Emmett. Molly had recommended the Seattle Care Cancer Alliance after being successfully treated for Hodgkin's lymphoma here.

At the beginning, all these minds are crucial. It takes that many of us to begin to understand what's happening.

Dr. Keith Eaton, my new oncologist who recently completed a research fellowship with the Fred Hutchinson Research Center, starts out by asking, "How much do you know about your condition?"

"Well, the biopsy surgeon said I had stage 4 cancer and it was inoperable, but we don't like him," I blurt out. We don't like him? I hear myself saying this as if his personality is relevant to the diagnosis.

"Well, we won't know what stage this is until we have some more test results," Dr. Eaton says. "I'm going to schedule you for a PET scan to see if the cancer has spread elsewhere in your body, and an MRI to see if it has gone to your brain."

It takes 90 seconds to complete the cycle in which stress chemicals are triggered, surge through the body, and then are flushed out of the blood stream[2]—which is a long time to not be thinking clearly while the doctor is still talking. At the words "spread elsewhere," I become the dog in the *Far Side* cartoon where the master has just given intricate instructions to "Go the door. Fetch my paper. Bring me my slippers, Rover," and all the dog hears is, "Blah, blah, blah, blah, Rover."

I look around the room. Kelly is shell-shocked. Camilla is steeling herself to stay present; Isaac is trying to get his head around it; Molly is being thrown back into her own diagnosis; Seth looks to be our only hope for objectivity. But we each have our 90-second cycles, so later on it will take all of us to recap what the doctor has said.

"If it is stage 3B, there are some things we can try," Dr. Eaton offers. "If it is stage 4 there is a promising clinical trial, but we'll have to see if there is enough tissue in your biopsy to test for the genetic mutation that would make you eligible for the trial." Clinical trial? That sounds good, doesn't it? But if the quality of the sample is dependent on the forethought of my biopsy surgeon, I'm not hopeful.

My advice to anyone facing a similarly terrifying conversation is this: Record it.

Why me?

A talented mystery writer I greatly admire once told me that I could start this story before the beginning, at the beginning, or after the beginning. For a cancer patient, it is impossible to know where the beginning is. Does it date back to a gene carried by my grandmother who died of lung cancer? Does it date back to a childhood of rolling in white fertilizer like it was fresh snow after my father had treated the lawn? Was it any combination of the 50,000 chemicals being used in the U.S. of which only a tiny fraction have been tested for carcinogenic effect?[3] Was it my previous cancer gone astray, or the hysterectomy I had in 2001 robbing me of protective hormones? Was it recent or chronic stress? Was it the absence or presence of something? Too much or too little? When is the fuse lit, and how long before the explosion?

Like a jilted lover, I could easily obsess over why my relationship with Life is ending and all the things I could have done differently. But it's a waste of time.

Dr. Eaton doesn't know the answers. I fall into none of the usual vectors: smoking, radon or asbestos exposure. With only one data point, he can only hazard a guess as to how long the disease has been growing inside me: four to five years. Dr. Eaton is comfortable with not knowing how this started, but his reluctance to come up with a cause is not shared by others. Everyone, it turns out—and I mean my hairdresser, too—has a theory. They fall into four categories:

- Well, no wonder, you're always working so hard (spoken compassionately). *Okay, but then why isn't everyone on the Microsoft campus already dead?*
- You eat too much junk (said judgmentally). *A lot of people eat a lot worse than I do and they're still healthy.*
- Must be unresolved issues with your past (said pensively). *Wouldn't that mean that all war vets with chronic post-traumatic stress would get cancer?*
- You haven't accepted Jesus into your life (said authoritatively). *Does any religion guarantee freedom from cancer? Show me the statistical backup, and I may join.*

We don't ask "why" when we get a cold or the flu (although we might point a finger at "who"), but because we're so scared of cancer we try to label it, stuff it in a box, and sit on the lid to keep the boogey man from popping out. In every lay theory of why cancer starts, there is an unstated, "So if I do this or don't do that, I won't get it. I will NOT get cancer." In my case this thought has its ironic side. The one thing everyone agrees on is that if you smoke you're at high risk for lung cancer.[4] The corollary would seem to be that if you don't smoke you aren't likely to get it. But I did get it—along with 20% of the women and 13% of the men with lung cancer who also never smoked.[5]

⊙ ⊙ ⊙

"It is stage 4," says Dr. Eaton. "I cannot cure you. And we don't have a big enough tissue sample to make you eligible for the trial. I can only offer palliative care."

There are no words to describe how it feels to be sitting at the edge of an examining room table being told I am going to die, and soon. Why? Because there is no *thing* to describe. I literally feel nothing. How did I end up in this room? How did my family end up here? They are showing signs of registering what is happening, but I'm sitting on the elevated examining table, my legs dangling, my mind in another universe altogether.

Medicine has come up short. Palliative? Does this mean a morphine haze? I struggle to draw meaning from my oncologist's words, as if I'm in the middle of a vocabulary test I forgot to study for. My PET scan shows a four-centimeter-by-six-centimeter mass in my left lung, and two smaller masses in my right. The cancer has spread to multiple lymph nodes in the middle of my chest. An ultrasound raises the possibility that the cancer has also spread to the liquid around my heart (called pericardial effusion). And my brain MRI shows three cancerous lesions there—proof of metastatic disease, which conclusively places me at stage 4.

I force myself to focus as Dr. Eaton says I don't look like his typical lung cancer patient. "You're still relatively healthy," he continues. "Let's keep you that way."

Dr. Eaton explains that neither surgery nor radiation are options for me, since the cancer has already spread. We could consider chemotherapy, but it would severely diminish my quality of life and probably not gain me much time. So instead he offers me a targeted therapy called Tarceva. The promise of the new world of targeted therapies is that they only block the activity of mutated cells, without incurring the collateral damage of traditional chemotherapy. But in 2006 it's largely an unfulfilled promise. Tarceva hasn't been shown to cure cancer; it merely keeps it from spreading further—and it doesn't work for everyone. In the 2004 Tarceva clinical trial, Asian women nonsmokers were the only group with any success.[6] Dr. Eaton hopes that because I meet two of those three qualifications I will respond. Dr. Eaton calls it a way to buy time while we wait for new drugs to come through the pipeline. So there's the definition of palliative care that my mind is still searching for.

What I don't fully appreciate is that Tarceva—a tablet the size of an aspirin I will take once a day for as long as it's effective—is not approved as a first line of defense against cancer. It's usually offered only to patients who have already taken traditional chemotherapy. Dr. Eaton is already getting creative. He is also willing to fight my insurance company to cover the cost of his unorthodox approach. (He will not only win the fight, in 2012, he will be proven right when Tarceva is shown to be a more effective than conventional chemotherapy for first-line treatment for patients with EGFR mutations.[7])

Although Dr. Eaton hates to be backed into a corner for a prognosis, we can't stop ourselves from asking. His estimate is a year—if the Tarceva works. (My primary physician told me much later that her statistical chart gave me only 3 months, due to the fluid surrounding my heart.) To address the brain tumors, Dr. Eaton immediately calls a radiation oncologist and colleague at the University of Washington, Dr. Jason Rockhill. Within the hour Dr. Rockhill is presenting us with my options at the UW Medicine Gamma Knife Center.

"We could continue to observe you. Given that you are starting Tarceva, we may see some response, however the brain is usually a sanctuary from systemic agents so this is unlikely. The second option is whole brain radiation. This has been the standard treatment for brain metastases for many decades. The advantage is it will treat not only the three lesions we see today but also any lesions that the MRI can't yet detect but which may be already present."

"What are the risks of whole-brain radiation?" I ask warily.

"Of most concern is the potential for long-term side effects such as difficulties with short-term memory, multitasking, and mood."

This sounds ghastly. "Do I have any other choice?" (Dr. Rockhill will write in my chart[8] that "she is in no apparent distress," but believe me, I am.)

"Yes, a reasonable option would be Gamma Knife, a form of highly-targeted radiation. To ensure accuracy, we would place a head frame on your skull. There is a remote chance of a skull fracture that could be life-threatening. Furthermore, there is the potential that we could identify new lesions on the treatment-planning MRI, which might make us proceed directly to whole brain radiation. But assuming no surprises, the potential side-effects are nausea, vomiting, fatigue, and headache."

"What about side-effects to how my brain works?"

"If there are any, we can manage them with steroids."

"How soon can you schedule me?"

"Next week."

I'm feeling healthy and strong, so it's hard to believe my condition is so dire—at least not until I read the What-You-Need-to-Know-About-Lung-Cancer-Before-You-Die booklet Dr. Eaton hands us at the end of the appointment. Then I realize I'm a goner. So what to do? Looks like I have a choice of lying here in the middle of this dark canyon I've fallen into, or getting up and walking.

CHAPTER TWO
Flickers of Hope

May, 2006

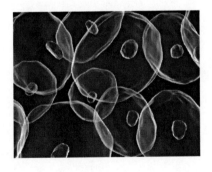

know that it is only my egocentrism that expects the whole world to turn gray when my thoughts get dark. Still, the view from our house of the Admiralty Inlet and the jagged Olympic Mountains is so breathtaking that I find myself unable to latch on to the idea that soon I may not be here to enjoy it. Friends hug me on the street and in stores, still wearing pink bracelets from the Love-In; family members always keep someone by my side. Life is too good for the diagnosis to be true. Yet this afternoon, as I walk up the steep hill behind the house with Thea in her sling, I feel terror as I struggle for breath. What if I won't live to see her grow up?

My inner world is equally disorienting. When I was forty I started psychotherapy. Sarri Gilman, my therapist, discovered that guided imagery was a good way for me to penetrate my emotional defenses. Images came easily to me and they felt honest—true reflections of my state of mind. During our three months of therapy I would spend the moments before our sessions sitting on the weathered staircase outside Sarri's office. I closed my eyes, relaxed, felt the sun on my face, and waited for an image to appear. This snapshot would be our starting point for the day. With the assistance of these images Sarri helped me move quickly to a place of integration and peace, and we ended our work together.

But a year later I had a dream that seemed significant, about discovering a recently deceased friend on a stretcher in my basement covered only by a thin, pink sheet. "But she doesn't belong there," I screamed to everyone, to no avail. When I told Sarri the details of the dream, she looked me in the eye and encouraged me to see a doctor.

The first doctor said, "It's nothing. The bleeding is from hemorrhoids; I can't see them but I'm sure they're there."

"No," I thought, "I had a dream."

The second doctor said, "I can't find anything, but I can run a test and get an answer to you in three weeks."

Three weeks? "What if the results are positive?" I asked.

"Again, I don't think they will be, but I would refer you to an internist."

I left her office and immediately scheduled an appointment with the internist, who felt a mass during the physical exam and sent me for definitive tests at the local hospital. They revealed a tumor in my rectum that was close to—but not quite—penetrating the rectal wall. A thin pink sheet of tissue was holding off metastasis.

So I don't know what to call these images, or this process I have of "seeing" them, but I do know to pay close attention to them.

Today the image of my lung as a woman with a boulder on her chest scares me. It corresponds so closely with the test results that I am afraid to let myself see what other terrors lie ahead. But after the MRI reveals I have brain cancer I lie down, still my mind, and wait for a new image to appear out of the blackness. I expect to see myself and two others: Lung Woman who I've met already, and Brain Woman who will reveal herself. But that's not what happens.

 The women who identified themselves as my organs are still gathered around me in a circle, but it is no longer night and there is no longer a helicopter in the distance. The women are tall, beautiful, and more uniformly shaped than women normally are. They are of heroic proportions. I am held by one of them in the middle of the circle, much like Mary holds Jesus in the Pietà, but I know I'm not dead yet because I can feel the other women beaming their healing light at me.

A profound shift has occurred since my last visualization. This story is no longer primarily about one organ, Lung Woman, it's about all of me: lungs, brain, and whatever else needs healing. And I am no longer the one offering help; I'm the one being helped. While it's true that I don't look so hot lying in the lap of the Madonna, at least the boulder is gone. I'm no longer flat on the tarmac. I'm better.

Who are these mythical women? They have identified themselves as my organ systems but I start calling them my goddesses. (I can't help it that my mother named me Diana, the Goddess of the Moon. Besides where is the power, mystery, and mythological ancestry in a healer called Pancreas Woman?) The next night, the goddesses call on me. We pick up where we left off, but this time I am able to sit up while I'm being held. Some of my own power seems to be coming back, but I've only been on Tarceva one day. Is this simply wishful thinking? God knows, I need some of that. Yet in the inner recesses of my mind, I don't call it wishful; I call it hope, even though I keep it to myself. Everyone knows me as a logical person; I'm not yet ready to disabuse them.

Within a week of starting holding my fingers and toes, Susan notices that I stop coughing during these Jin Shin Jyutsu "treatments." So now whenever I start to cough, someone rushes over to gently grasp my big toe and pinky finger. Everyone is drafted: nephews, nieces, children, children-in-law, friends who walk in the door, and skeptically at first, but most importantly, Kelly.

I'm relieved that we've finally found something everyone can do to help. At first we sit self-consciously close to each other on our comfortable couch, making jokes about the smell of my feet. (I keep my socks on.) We make small talk, the nervous chatter of those who have never done anything this woo-woo before, but we quickly become fascinated. I can feel how distinct each person's energy is, and I'm starting to feel something happening in my body during the treatments, although I can't quite describe it yet.

The holders feel something as well, a beat or pulse in each finger and toe that usually starts off out of rhythm with the others but then synchronizes.

But what we feel in our fingers is no match for what we feel for each other in our hearts: in this moment, no one else in the world matters.

I Think You Ought to Book Your Travel Now...

This is what they tell you when you've got stage 4 cancer: prepare for the worst, expect the best, and book your travel now. In Dr. Eaton's view, I will never be stronger than I am in this moment. Now would be the time to fulfill that life dream, whatever it is. But in *my* view of my future, I'm *not* going to steadily decline. I'm going to heal, and I don't want anything to get in the way of it—not exhaustion from travel, nor virulent bugs from far-off places, nor viruses caught en route. So what to put on the Top 10 List now that Life has politely asked me to quit procrastinating and fill that list out?

Sitting with my pencil and paper, I can only come up with three things:

1. Be with family and friends that live nearby.
2. Visit family that lives farther away. (It seems there's no destination in the world more important than the one called family.)

So what's number 3? I call our friend, Randy, who we've walked with every Sunday for fifteen years.

"Randy, I know what I want to do before I die," I say.

"Georgia," Randy calls out to his wife (also my good friend), "Could we make an exception to our wedding vows for a dying woman?"

"Not *that*, Randy," I laughingly interject.

"Oh. Well, the only other thing I can imagine is that you want to sing with the Rural Characters," he allows, without missing a beat. The Rural Characters is the local band that sang at the Love-In. Its members sing of our community, make light of our trials, and honor those of us who need honoring. On the spur of the moment Randy graciously creates a Rural Characters Adopt-A-Wish Foundation to allow me to sing in their annual concert next week.

The two-hour rehearsal is blissful. The sound of acoustic guitars, a mandolin, bucket bass, ukuleles, concertina, and sixteen voices reverberates throughout the hand-timbered room. I edge my voice in the direction of a deep alto, feeling our spirits merge together as effortlessly as our voices find the harmony. I will later read studies of how people's heart and brain rhythms synchronize when they make music together, but right now I don't need science to back up this feeling. Over the years singing has helped me bond with family, build lifelong friendships, court my husband, raise my children, and soothe my grandchildren. When I put my headphones on later that night, I allow the music to flow through me in hopes of connecting to the twenty-one-year-old music major that loved it so much. I want to find her, that girl I was, for she lived fully, had the stamina of a dancer, the invincibility of youth, and the resilience to constantly adapt to change. If somewhere along the line a single gene had mutated in the generations of cells shaped by love, marriage, family, service, work, travel, success, failure, exhilaration, resignation, and exposure to toxins, wasn't she the one to lead me back to health?

Igniting The Promise of Hope

When I wake up today, it feels like there's no way back to health at all. It's blocked by a brick wall of grief. Our 25-year-old son, Eric, and his wife, Kylie, have just flown in from her brother's wedding. They will stay until the Gamma Knife procedure, but will have to return to their home and work in Indiana shortly after. Seeing them, holding them, I can't bear to think how few my days with them will be.

Both Eric and Kylie are sorry to have missed the Love-In but their late arrival turns out to be fortuitous, for they have also missed the doctors' appointments. They have not yet been overwhelmed by the white coats. They have hope in their eyes as they sit on the edge of the ottoman in our living room looking up at me. I'm pacing, not daring to sit down for fear that I'll need to quickly escape upstairs to cry. They've just handed me what they call the Granny Dinani Healing Plan—a list of foods I should take out of my diet and new foods I should include.

"Mom, of all people, you can do it," Eric says, with Kylie nodding in agreement.

They call it determination; I call it naïveté. Don't you get it? I want to tell them. Don't you see that there is no magic bullet here? There is no one food or supplement that will turn this tide. I've lived long enough to see many miracle cancer cures fall flat.

But Eric and Kylie, though young, are not naïve. Seven months earlier, Kylie too was diagnosed with a serious illness that doctors cannot yet cure. Her immune system is overactive and mine is underactive, but we both need to understand how that system works and what we can do to influence it. And what Eric and Kylie are recommending is no fad. Dr. Andrew Weil, a pioneer in the now widely accepted field of integrative medicine, inspired the two of them to manage her illness by changing their diet and lifestyle.

They give me Weil's *Spontaneous Healing* to inspire me to harness the body's natural healing power, and *8 Weeks to Optimum Health* to give me some specific ideas on how to do that.

"You can do it, Mumsy."

They may have saved my life. That night, I read Dr. Weil's book huddled in bed with the covers wrapped tightly around me. "Healing is a natural power,"[9] he writes. "DNA has within it all the information needed to repair itself."[10] Weil says that healing is spontaneous in the sense that the body automatically takes on the job of fixing the body's structural damage. My contractor had fallen down on the job, I think, either because my body hadn't recognized the damage or wasn't up to the repair. Weil himself seems to agree with my assessment; his final chapter talks about cancer and how it represents a "significant failure of the healing system," and that spontaneous remission was an "all-too-rare event."

Weil writes of a mind/body connection that could activate our natural healing system. But how am I going to do that? By closing my eyes, clicking the heels of my ruby red slippers, and saying, "There's no place like hope, there's no place like hope?" It turns out that Weil's message is much more powerful—and practical. Our bodies are built to heal themselves; it's what they do. We are all natural healers. Although we've grown used to outsourcing to doctors, our innate capabilities can be strengthened, much the way we do our muscles and our minds. Weil recommends many things that make sense to me, which I soon adopt: good diet, exercise, and dramatic changes in lifestyle to minimize stress and healing on all levels—physical, mental, emotional, and spiritual.

It doesn't hurt to try.

But perhaps it is telling that one of the post-its I leave in the book flags the following observation: "Denial is a natural anesthetic, and while it has a bad reputation (of course, it is unhealthy if it persists), it may be very useful as a temporary mechanism to permit a basic level of functioning when the full impact of the grief would be devastating."[11]

I have no training in meditation. I don't do yoga. For the past years, I've been eating on the fly, exercising infrequently and sleeping poorly. I've been listening to the demands of my job more than my body. Weil says I can find the mind/body connection by paying attention to my breathing but all this does is remind me that my breath is short and my terror is wide.

But it wasn't always this way. In addition to loving music, I also used to be a dancer and choreographer. I knew what it was like to enter what famous choreographer Twyla Tharp calls the white room of my mind and wait for inspiration. During my dance career that inspiration usually came under the pressure of a deadline. My prognosis was equally effective.

And I'm not the only one. The ability of imagery to emerge spontaneously from within us is just part of what our brains do. It's not guided, nor intentional; it doesn't come from current sensory input. It can seem like simply the random processing of all the thoughts, images, sounds, and smells of the day. But when I can get my mind still, if only for an instant, when I can recall my conscious mind from its propensity to take over my entire brain and allow it to retreat to its place as just *one part* of my brain, then there's an opportunity for something significant to emerge. An "aha." A new understanding. A creative thought. A snap judgment. A moment where my mind synthesizes all it knows, strips away the non-essential in order to reveal what is essential, and then it wants to let me know what it knows.

In the dance studio, this communication was in the form of dance phrases. So far, with this cancer, my mind is serving up ancient Greek pageantry but it's effective; I am good at reading body language so this gestural imagery is easy for me to understand. So tonight I quiet myself with some classical music and return to my visualization where I left off the night before. Each night the story seems to unfold on the same stage, one scene, one brief snapshot at a time. I stand up. I lift my arms to the light. I spin joyously.

The images show me getting stronger, yet I've only been on Tarceva a week. Dr. Eaton said it would be three weeks before I would experience all the side effects, and he gave me no hope that Tarceva would ever restore me to health. So I interpret the imagery as a reflection of my rising spirit. Of my determination to survive. Of the decision to take charge of my own healing.

The reclusive poet Emily Dickenson once referred to hope as a "thing with feathers that ... never stops at all, and ... never, in extremity, it asked a crumb of me." That's a nice sentiment, but with all due respect, Emily should have gotten out more. This is not my experience of hope. Hope stops often. It asks daily, and sometimes every minute, to be tended like a fire. Hope begins like the first strike of a match, a flicker of flame that only survives if it is quickly fed just the right tinder.

For me, the first shred of newspaper held to that flame was the moment my niece, Jessie, told me about a friend's mother with stage 4 cancer that went into remission. Another wad of newspaper was the comment from Dr. Eaton that I was "stronger than his typical patient," along with my primary doctor's observation that "You must have a strong immune system if you're living life at full blast with stage 4 cancer because most people would be flat out in bed." With Granny Dinani's Healing Plan backed by Andrew Weil's books, Eric and Kylie provided the first substantial piece of kindling. My visualizations are contributing the second.

The Other 1% Club

For a lung cancer patient, the Internet is not a friendly place. Unlike breast cancer sites that feature smiling, happy women running triathlons, the lung cancer sites I visit are filled with sermons about smoking. Perhaps this is because there isn't any good news about lung cancer. While 89% of breast cancer patients will survive at least five years, the odds drop to only 15% for lung cancer patients[12]—and these are mostly patients diagnosed at stage I. The website I'm reading tells me that the equivalent of three jumbo jets filled with American lung cancer patients die every day.

I quickly shut down my computer, but I feel like I'm trying to undo knowing someone has died. At my next appointment I ask Dr. Eaton what my odds are of living to see Thea in kindergarten.

"Only 1% survive for five years,"[13] he answers.

That was yesterday. Today I'm wondering, "So how do I get into the 1% Club?" In May 2006, no one has an answer for that. That's the thing about this 1% Club: the rules for joining are unknown. If they were widely available, it would be called the 80% Club.

I slump. I pick myself back up. Give myself a pep talk. Membership is improbable but it is not impossible. It is not the 0% Club. I've been in the 1% Club before. I was a good student; my husband and I created and partnered a small business that has been successful for 17 years and counting. What are the odds of that? But I don't think my lung cancer cells are evaluating my ability to perform well on a standardized test, or to make a strong marketing pitch. So I continue to think about probabilities. I'm the only one with my genes, my history, my thoughts, my loves, my joys, my despairs, my exposure to toxins, and my supply of what feeds me, which means I'm actually in the 1-in-6.5 Billion Club. So it should be a cinch to find my way into the 1-in-a-100 Club.

What's the meaning of a statistic anyway? This particular statistic means that in any population of one hundred people, ninety-nine do things the same way (and die), and one does things differently (and lives). The message is clear: it's time to find some ideas outside of what most people agree is reasonable. If I'm asking Dr. Eaton to challenge his assumptions about the fate of lung cancer patients, why not challenge my own assumptions about healing being the exclusive provenance of doctors and pharmaceuticals?

If Tarceva and I get along, I probably won't be weakened by it like I might have been by traditional chemotherapy; low blood counts won't keep me away from friends and family. *I, as a patient, am now free to fully participate in my healing from cancer.* My doctors have said, metaphorically, that they can't get me from Seattle to New York, but they are also saying they'll take me as far as they can. I'm grateful for every mile and every tank of gas they have to give. I just don't know whether it's going to get me to Denver or New Jersey, but since I want to go farther than Tarceva is likely to take me it's up to me to find other ways to cover the remaining distance.

But how will I know whether the 1% ideas I find will be good for me? Without adequate scientific evidence how can I keep from falling prey to any crackpot scheme that comes along? Well, let's get real: What do I have to lose? My pride? Expendable. Our cash? We'll spend it carefully. My health? I won't put my faith in any substance, natural or not, that could conceivably interfere with Tarceva's inner chemistry, and we'll take it from there.

So line 'em up. Tarceva, how much are you in for? In the phase III clinical trial that led to this drug's FDA approval, the median of patients on Tarceva showed only a two-month survival gain—from 4.7 to 6.7 months—compared to those on placebo.[14] Hmm. Not enough. After one year, 31 percent of patients taking Tarceva were still alive compared to 22 percent of those taking the placebo. It's good to hear that some patients were living longer than a year, but hold on, what's this placebo effect?

It turns out that since the 1950s, every clinical trial has had to adjust for the astonishing power of the placebo effect[15]—if you believe a medical intervention will work, it will. Subsequently, researchers have discovered the nocebo effect[16]—if you don't believe it will work, it won't. So that's significant: I'll be as open as I possibly can to believing things will help. It turns out that hope itself heals by releasing endorphins and enkephalins—neurotransmitters that were discovered to be linked to the immune system back in 1987.[17]

Who else? What else? Where else? A friend sent an email about me to Dr. Weil, who actually responded! "Tell her to try Vitamin D (2,000 mg/day), Host Defense mushrooms (with Zhu Ling), and melatonin so she can sleep."

Vitamin D for cancer? Okay. How effective are you, Vitamin D? How many tanks of gas are you good for?

Mushrooms? It sounds crazy, but the Chinese studies I find claim improvements as high as 50%.[18] ("The studies aren't up to our burden of proof," says Dr. Eaton, "but there are metastudies in the Western literature that indicate more research is warranted. And it won't hurt the Tarceva.")

Studies show social support improves survival, too.[19] How do you measure the power of the Love-In?

Can I just start adding up all these numbers and hope I can make it at least as far as the first pass over the Cascade Mountains? (You're shaking your head. Statistics don't work that way, you're thinking. Probably not, but the truth is, right now statistics don't work for me at all, so I'm going to keep adding them up until I'm counted out.)

In this moment Gamma Knife is my best medical shot at buying time. Untreated, brain cancer can kill in two months. But the procedure is still a week away, and I can start working on myself right now.

Fighting Fire With Fire: Gamma Knife

The Gamma Knife utilizes a technique called stereotactic radiosurgery, which uses multiple beams of radiation converging in three dimensions to focus precisely on a small volume, such as a tumor, permitting intense doses of radiation to be delivered to that volume safely.[20]

I am going to have 201 beams focused on each of the three lesions of my brain. Each beam is harmless on its own and only gets enough power to destroy the lesion by intersecting with the other 200 in a single, tiny location. This precision gives me a chance of avoiding collateral damage to my healthy brain cells. I am very eager to keep every one I can. I am terrified of losing any of my ability to think and feel (although right now temporary amnesia could come in handy).

Under local anesthesia, a special rigid head frame incorporating a three-dimensional coordinate system is attached to the patient's skull with four screws.

Ouch. One neurosurgeon says to three medical students, "Ready everyone, shoot the Novocaine! Ready, everyone, screw!"

Camilla, Isaac, Eric, and Kylie see the humor in that and everything else, as they take on the job of keeping me laughing for four hours while I wait with them in pre-op with a metal cage screwed into my head.

Kel is waiting with Thea in the waiting room because she's not allowed inside. He covers her eyes as Art, the nurse, wheels me past them and down the hallway to get the MRI they will use to target the radiation. Art starts humming *I Got Rhythm*, which happens to be one of the songs in the Broadway musical *Crazy for You* that I directed for Eric's high school. I still remember all the words so we sing them in full voice as we roll down the dark basement corridor, with the gurgling plumbing pipes overhead and squeaky wheelchair providing accompaniment.

When we get to the elevator, the other three people waiting to get on do their best not to look my way.

"Do you like my party hat?" I ask the tall lanky guy.

"No, I don't, and I hope I never have to wear one," he says as kindly as he can while shuddering.

I hope so too.

Imaging studies, such as magnetic resonance imaging (MRI), are then obtained and the results are sent to the Gamma Knife's planning computer system.

Dr. Rockhill talks briefly with Kel as he passes through the waiting room on his way to consult with his colleagues in the planning area. He then comes into my room and pulls up both today's scans and last week's on two different monitors.

"Great news. There are only two lesions," he announces to me and the kids.

"What happened to the third?" we ask simultaneously.

"We don't know," he says. He shows us where the three lesions were on the original MRI and where the current two are located. I ask him which areas of the brain he will be targeting.

"Multi-tasking and left-side coordination," he responds.

The multi-tasking answer draws an immediate laugh. After running a company, raising children, and directing plays in my spare time, I'm the person everyone figures can lose some multi-tasking ability and still end up normal. We don't talk about the left-side coordination. For someone who loves to dance as much as I do, losing any functionality here would be tough.

Together, physicians and medical radiation physicists routinely consider numerous fine-tuning adjustments of treatment parameters until an optimal plan and dose are determined.

While we're waiting, the four family members in the room

give me a fingers-and-toes Jin Shin treatment. Camilla is last. As she begins to touch me, I go into meditation:

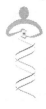

We are inside a soccer ball lined with hexagonally-shaped cells. One of the goddess-like figures from the first meditation carefully extracts the cancerous cells and moves them into the center of the ball, preparing them to be irradiated. She then methodically coats each of the remaining healthy cells with a thick blue gel to protect them from radiation.

I feel very calm and confident after this vision, and my blood pressure and stress are low as a result.

Using the three-dimensional coordinates determined in the planning process, the frame is then precisely attached to the Gamma Knife unit to guarantee that when the unit is activated, the target is placed exactly in the center of approximately 200 precision-aimed, converging beams of (Cobalt-60 generated) gamma radiation.

I am the target. I am bolted into the machine. Stay calm, Diana. There is nowhere to run, nowhere to hide.

But there is.

Inside my mind there is no metal frame, no giant beam of radiation. The playlist Eric and Kylie have made relaxes me. And while normally these songs would trigger memories of special family occasions, today the songs are an invitation for my family to hold my hand during the GammaKnife room in the protected area of my mind—Kelly, our children, my parents and parents in-law, my siblings and siblings-in-law, and all of my nieces and nephews, each in turn show up to dance with me in this inner studio. It feels real, timeless, and euphoric but when my head starts to heat up from the radiation I need more help to stay in the meditative state.

Suddenly an image of Kelly and me with our grandchildren pops into my head and makes me so intensely curious that that the radiology technician has to tell me twice that the session is over.

Grandchildren? We only have one. But in this meditation, there are three of them.

"You did beautifully," says the technician. "All of your vitals were great." For the second time that day, I have hints that what happens in my mind impacts my body.

Following treatment the headframe is removed and the patient may return to normal activity.

"Can I sing tonight?" I ask, feeling nothing but soreness from the frame.

"I'd like you to stay close to the hospital tonight in case you need to come back in," says Dr. Rockhill.

"Tomorrow?"

"Tomorrow you can sing."

And I do, onstage with the Rural Characters at the Whidbey Island Center for the Arts. The warmth coming from all the family and friends in the audience, the exhilaration of singing harmonies, and the magic of bringing Thea backstage, could have easily earned this night its place on the Bucket List. But it is bucking the cancer—standing on my own power under the hot array of stage lights, singing lyrics my brain can still remember even though it's just been blasted by gamma rays, demonstrating my resilience in front of my children to help lessen their fear—that blazes this night into my soul.

⊙ ⊙ ⊙

The Love-in, leaving our business, the tests, the waiting, the results: they're all catching up with us. We have had unflagging support, which means that the house has been full. Little Thea running around has brought both joy and chaos. And Kel has been by my side every second.

The day after the concert all is silent. The house has cleared out for the afternoon and Kelly and I are alone together, too exhausted to say a word. We slump onto opposing couches, books in hand, when the phone rings. My mother wants to know how the Gamma Knife treatment went, and about those three lesions that mysteriously became two. "Maybe Tarceva," I say, although the doctor didn't think so. "Maybe it's the visualizations!" I tell my mother, with a tiny glimmer of hope in my voice.

I hang up and smile at the man I love. He says, "Is that the story you want to tell people? Because it's okay if you do, I just want to be sure I've got it straight, so we're saying the same thing."

He's talking to me with what he believes is compassion, but I feel as if he's just punched me in the gut. And I react. "What do you mean 'the same story?' Weren't you there? Didn't you hear Dr. Rockhill?"

"I heard him to say they might have misinterpreted the first MRI," he says.

"Dr. Rockhill showed us the two scans side by side after he talked with you in the waiting room and there were clearly three lesions on the first MRI and two on the second. Are you saying that I'm just kidding myself? This is my only hope! How can you not support me?" I snap.

And this poor man who has been on the ragged edge of losing his life partner for two weeks now, who cannot sleep and can barely hide his tears, is undone that I would think he is not supporting me. He withdraws upstairs. I follow him. We have been here before in our marriage. He's profoundly hurt and doesn't want to talk about it, and I'm hurt and do want to talk about it. He escapes from the house and drives aimlessly around Whidbey Island in no state of mind to be behind the wheel.

I can't take this, not on top of everything else. So when Kelly returns late that night I tell him—not ask him—that we have to go to see my therapist, Sarri. He has never wanted to do this, he doesn't believe in therapy. But he loves me. And he goes.

Sarri does not take on our marriage. She does not take on what did or didn't happen with Dr. Rockhill or with each other. She knows Kel is hurting but she's doing triage. She simply says, "The only person whose story really counts right now is Diana. She's the one who has to find hope inside herself. It is her body that needs to believe. Everyone else's story may be right, but hers is the only one that matters."

At least this is what I hear. My mind starts spinning around Sarri's acknowledgement that my hope might be strung together by the slenderest of threads. In the relative safety of her presence I let myself feel how precarious my situation is and how it requires all of my energy to hold myself together. So I don't recognize the implications of Kel's question back to Sarri:

"But then who do I talk to?"

"Someone else," she says. "Tom, Miles, Randy, one of your other friends."

I don't register that for Kelly sharing his fears with those close to both of us seems treasonous. I don't realize that he feels like he's already lost me emotionally, because now he can't share his feelings with me.

I am so desperately trying to get purchase on the wall of the cliff that I don't see Kelly free-falling over the edge.

A Change in Command

If I can fire myself from my own company, surely I can get rid of the clamor from the left side of my brain and turn leadership over to the quieter inner voice on my right. I have spent my whole life dancing back and forth across my corpus callosum between what Daniel Pink in his book, *A Whole New Mind,* calls "Left-brain-Directed Thinking"—sequential, literal, functional, textual, and analytic—and "Right brain-Directed Thinking"—simultaneous, metaphorical, aesthetic, contextual, and synthetic[21] (as in *synthesis,* not *polyester*). At the time of my diagnosis, I was in a very L-directed career as president of a marketing consulting company. I had had enough L-directed education to get two degrees from Stanford University. But my training in the arts had given me skills in creativity, synthesis, and flexibility that are the hallmarks of the right brain and these were relevant far beyond the dance studio. I was good at analyzing any business process, but our success as a company rode on my ability to pull many visions and ideas into a single whole that we could then embrace and collaborate on.

Now I am ready to hand over full command to the right part of my brain. I have already outsourced L-directed thinking to some of the best medical and scientific minds in the country—and they still don't have an answer. I don't think I could do better by giving myself a crash course in molecular biology. I know that the right brain is where my creative centers are and intuitively I believe this might be where the healing centers are. Given that the autonomic system is unconscious, perhaps I could get closer to it by exploring other parts of my brain than my conscious mind. But before I can fully embrace allowing the right side of my brain to take over, I have to appease my left side, the majority party that just lost the election. In a last grab at waning power, they put me in front of their subcommittee and grill me.

Has this mind/body connection stuff ever really helped anybody?

Come on, we've already been through this. We read Andrew Weil, and Bernie Siegel's *Love, Medicine, and Miracles,* and Norman Cousin's *Anatomy of an Illness* when we got cancer the first time. We know that Dr. Carl Simonton and his wife Stephanie[22] had success with cancer patients using visualization and guided imagery.

Yes, but did they say anything about stage 4 lung cancer?

Irrelevant question. This is what we've got, so we've got to work with it.

If your precious immune system is so all-powerful, how did you get into this mess in the first place?

Our bodies successfully fight cancer all the time; it's just that once a tumor gets to a certain size, it coats itself with a protein that disguises it, becoming a wolf in sheep's clothing. By the time it's recognized as a problem, the tumor may be in a position to overwhelm the immune system.

What makes you think your conscious mind can make a difference now?

I'm hoping my focused intention on healing will send a biological signal to my immune system patrols to go back into the lung neighborhood previously judged safe, and have another look.

Well then, if your mind can fight cancer, then your mind must have caused it.

(This question almost makes me give up, but I rally.) This is false logic. That the mind can help in healing does not mean the mind caused the illness. A leads to B leads to C does not mean that C leads to B. Dr. Candace Pert, the internationally-celebrated researcher in the mind/body connection, says "Specific types of dispositions, *e.g.,* 'fighting spirit' will slow the *course of cancer*, but the data is entirely clear that the *cause* of most cancer is environmental toxins, not anything we are thinking, feeling or believing (and not our genes)."[23]

Just because someone else has used the mind/body connection successfully doesn't mean you can find it and do anything with it.
Well, I'm already talking to Lung Woman and the goddesses...

Come on, Diana. Goddesses? Really?
Look, it's my body, so it's my language. And I've seen results. I'm getting stronger and my cough is weaker. The Tarceva is working better than Dr. Eaton expected, and what about that missing brain lesion?

What if you screw this up?
How can I possibly screw this up worse than it is already? Stage 4 cancer is pretty much the definition of "screwed up." (Composing myself, I continue.) My immune system knows more than I ever will about how it works, so I'm going to trust it and not worry about directing the conversation. In fact, I'm going to get out of the way. And now it's time for you to get out of the way, too.

With that, I usher in a new administration, one willing to work on solving the problem instead of bemoaning it with the same old litany.

⊙ ⊙ ⊙

I immediately start to see changes in my imagery. Instead of goddess-like figures drawn to human scale, there are now highly miniaturized and talented dancers actively working on the cancer cells on the surface of my lung. Instead of a seeing a single snapshot each night, the imagery has evolved to something more like a

YouTube clip. I'm now watching an ongoing dance on an inner healing stage.

Music is the main reason I can stay in this inner world so long. While listening to a Brahms Concerto, for example, I can lose myself in the dancers without my attention wandering off into what we're going to have for dinner, or how long it will take for the cancer to incapacitate me. Music is my Sherpa guide into this uncharted territory of my right brain[24] where I hope to find the centers of healing. And it turns out that because music predates language, the centers that help us assimilate and process music *are* spread throughout the brain. According to Daniel Levitin, professor of psychology and neuroscience at McGill University, music also lights up the same parts of the brain that trigger the chemicals for joy and love—and perhaps most importantly for me right now, for the placebo effect.[25] Music by itself has been shown to boost the immune system; one mechanism is by increasing the amount of immunoglobulin A, a critical antibody.[26]

Classical music works best for me because it has no words to distract me, and its variety of themes and moods keeps the dancers inventive.

The dancers are no longer limited by conventional reality— they can dance anywhere and be any size. Right now their stage is the surface of my left lung; the set is an expansive cave, contoured like the inner lining of my lung cavity, an arc with plenty of light below but undefined shadows above.

The dancers are having a blast. Working collectively like members of a hive, they are enthusiastically popping what looks like bubble wrap on the stage floor. A muscular male dancer throws in a high leap simply for the fun of it, and sticks the landing. In oncoming rows, dancers run, slide,

and stomp the floor, methodically working their way across
the surface of the floor.

When Kelly and I see Twyla Tharp's ballet *In the Upper Room* a few months later, I elbow him. "That's it! That's what it looks like! Those are my dancers." (I just didn't give them those cool red toe shoes.) But my dancers looked like they were having even more fun than Tharp's professionals, perhaps because my inner dancers realize that this is not just another show, another gig. There's a life at stake.

A few weeks later I'm surfing the web—still avoiding the lung cancer sites—but interested in learning more about targeted therapy. I know that based on current research, scientists hope that Tarceva will prevent tumor proliferation; they don't expect it to kill the tumor cell outright. Now I'm finding out why. Tarceva is an epidermal growth factor receptor (EGFR) *inhibitor*. Its job is to fly through the body and find one specific type of receptor on a lung cancer cell that, when mutated, signals the cell to grow uncontrollably; Tarceva tries to plug up the receptor before an energy molecule known as ATP can dock and deliver its payload. The dancers have it right in this meditation: it's all about making contact and stomping in.

I've been playing the Bach Brandenburg Concertos and fast-forwarding through the slow movements. My hard-working dancers want to keep moving quickly, to get the most work done. But one evening that starts to change.

Instead of a cast of hundreds of dancers, there is only one
dancer onstage. She is the woman that first picked me up
off the tarmac. I think of her as my immune system, but she
is more than that. She represents the totality of my healing

> *capacity. When she starts dancing to a haunting adagio she looks like Tandy Beal, my beautiful colleague from my days as a college dance instructor in Santa Cruz. There is nothing mournful in her movements, just sheer power. She reaches slowly through space in an arc, carving out the entire tumor, raising it high and releasing it joyfully.*

I remember from dance class how much more difficult it is to dance slowly than quickly: the dancer's powerful arabesque is an expression of my own strength and flexibility. When she slices space with her arms she is carving out time for me to be with my family. When she raises her arms high, she confidently lifts her chest to life—and suspends there.

☉ ☉ ☉

Tarceva may not be as harsh as conventional chemotherapy but it is not without its side effects, and three weeks into treatment they arrive right on schedule. So far I've kept my long hair, but I have an acne-like rash all over my face. That's what comes of wishing you could look young again. Then I have red and itchy zits all over my chest followed by a rash from my throat to my knees. And then all the rashes disappear. Thanks to Tarceva, I spend countless hours in the restroom at Barnes & Noble (3 stalls), Borders (up to 4), McDonalds (2 stalls), and anywhere else (1 stall=risky). I ask to see a nutritionist who gives me food choices to manage the symptoms but doesn't give me any guidance on foods that contribute to defeating the cancer.

I don't overwhelm my friends with details, but whenever any of this gets to be too much, I remember what Dr. Eaton said: "We think that those who experience the most side-effects initially do the best in the long run." And when Dr. Eaton mounts today's CT on the viewer and compares it to my first one, it looks like my run will be longer than predicted. My sister-in-law sends out the email while we all celebrate.

To: The support team
From: Susan Lindsay
Date: May 26, 2006
Subject: Diana update

WOW! The doctor took one look at the CTs and said, "Wow! Diana, I just want you to know that this is not the usual course. You are one of the lucky ones. I knew by looking at you, before I saw the CT, that the medicine was working, but this is not usual, not usual at all."

Dr. Eaton was stunned as we looked at the two sets of CTs, one from 4 weeks ago when Diana was first diagnosed, and the one from today. The first one looked like there was a gloved hand stretching across her lung, filmy, white, and ominous. In the second the tumor has shrunk by almost half!

Thanks to everyone for your thoughts, prayers, cards, emails, gifts, and support. A huge thank-you to the Lindsay Communications office for allowing Diana to rest and focus all her energy on the healing.

Love to all!
Susan

CHAPTER THREE

Opening Life's Medicine Cabinet

June–July, 2006

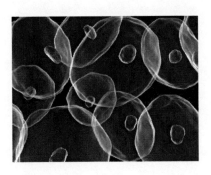

I t will be months before we know whether Gamma Knife has been effective because the resulting scar tissue looks the same as an untreated lesion on an MRI. Dr. Rockhill's benchmark for success is no further growth of the two treated lesions. However, suspecting that the cancer is still present in the brain in amounts too small to be detected by the MRI, he schedules bi-monthly scans in case he needs to play whack-a-mole with an emerging tumor. Dr. Eaton hopes that the Tarceva will provide me a few more months before developing resistance, and he scans me monthly to be sure he doesn't need to change his game plan. They are both playing defense.

Now that I know the worst symptoms of Tarceva, I'm ready to go on offense. I'm ready to take on the self-appointed job of rebuilding my immune system. I remember a study on leadership that suggested leaders focus first on the strengths of their organization, not the weaknesses. So what are mine?

1. I have *love* all around me—Kel, our children, grandchildren, my extended family, and the Whidbey Island community who surrounded us at the Love-In.
2. I have a strong *medical team.*
3. I have found a language to begin an *inner conversation.*
4. I have an appetite for *joy* and a way to create it in most situations.
5. I have the *intelligence* to understand what my doctors and my research are telling me.
6. I have the *creativity* to consider some off-the-beaten-path solutions.
7. I have the right *genetic mutation,* apparently, because Tarceva is starting to work.
8. I have *spirit*—a connectedness to nature and others; it's

not a religion, but a belief in forces larger than myself.

9. I have some financial *resources* and Kelly and I are willing to commit any or all of them to healing. We have a decent insurance policy (we hope), some cash savings, and retirement funds we could use, although I worry that this will jeopardize Kel's future.

10. I have the *resilience* to keep trying.

If these are my strengths, then what keeps them charged up? What keeps me tied to this earth and this life? I'm not sure yet, but I do know that this is my body, and it's my disease, so it will need to be my way of healing. We are not standard-issue colanders, each stamped with identical holes. What would fill up Diana? I'm not looking for a long-term answer. I'm looking for my next step.

What if I listen to my quiet voice, my inner compass, and simply ask it one question: *Do I feel better* doing this activity, thinking this thought, having this energy around, being in this moment? Does it help me find joy, and strengthen my will to live? If my body says "yes," I'll do it some more and keep exploring this avenue. But if my body says "no," well, first I'll consider the source. If this is the lazy part of me that doesn't want to get off the couch and take a walk, I'll override it. But if the "no" comes from a clear inner voice, I commit to stop doing whatever I'm doing.

So my body and I start walking together—forward, sideways, and sometimes in opposite directions because we are learning. My intuition grows—listening, trying, listening, trying—and my plan starts to unfold. I build hope every day; I practice healing.

The first steps are out the door and up the hill, with Thea wrapped in the sling around my body. What delights me is that I don't have to fly overseas for an exotic cure, or eat a diet that would repel everyone at the table. I'm focusing on the things right around me that make me feel best. Dr. Larry Dossey's book, *The Extraordinary Healing Power of Ordinary Things,* inspires me to look into the broader medicine cabinet of life. I begin to consider that the love, laughter, song, and dance that had made me feel better during the Love-In might in fact be protocols worth adding to the Tarceva regimen.

This is *my* path, not a prescription for anyone else, nor is it based on any belief system, including my own. This isn't even really about cancer, it's about healing my life.

Recapturing the Joy

If I'm going to heal my life, I need to start with the love of my life.

Every marriage has a story, a shared understanding of the plot line, at least at first. Ours is a love story. We still cuddle together all night long, hold hands while we stroll, sizzle when we dance, and even shower together in the morning. The last words we hear at night are "I love you sweetie," or "I love you, too."

But the last few years we have also been through the part of the plot "in which our hero and heroine face trials." Thanks largely to Thea, Kel recently emerged from what he refers to as his "Black and Blue" period, a depression that neither of us recognized as a disease. We didn't know what caused it any more than we know what caused my cancer. He believed it was work related, but I took it personally when I couldn't lift him out of it, which left both of us feeling confused, powerless, and occasionally angry. Now we both want to make up for lost time, for lost passion and compassion, but given my prognosis we're worried that we might not have a chance to do it. We leap at Sarri's suggestion to spend some time alone together.

We've booked a room in a Seattle hotel. We are here to walk it out, not talk it out. We wander the streets, hand in hand, corner after corner, for hours. We declare amnesty on the past with our first step outside. In a 1970s essay, biologist Lewis Thomas recalled that the root of the word "error" is "err," one meaning of which is "to wander." He figured that sometimes it took a lot of wandering before you got to the truth of a situation.[27] Somehow through 30 years of marriage, Kel and I had wandered off track, and so had my body. Now he and I stitch our hearts together again, just like we used to knit double mittens during our four-month honeymoon in Vermont, so we could go for walks together hand in hand, warm and protected against the freezing elements.

$$\odot \odot \odot$$

I'm continuing to check off my bucket list by flying to the East Coast to see my mother, my brother Cliff, my sister Annie, and their families. Three weeks after beginning Tarceva, I'm starting to feel better, but my family hasn't witnessed my resilience, and they still fear the worst.

Now that we're together I sense that my siblings are wondering whether every moment with me is the last one—the last steak-frites Cliff will cook for me, the last Beatles sing-a-long with my harmony added, the last hike in the woods sharing confidences with Annie and my siblings-in-law Carol and Doug, and the last performance by a niece or nephew I will ever see. Annie's in constant tears, Cliff is stoic. My mother sits with her hands perched on her lap insisting I will meet this challenge as I have all the others. She calls it "confidence in Diana;" the rest of the family calls it denial, and it's an easier target for everyone's feelings than my prognosis.

Once we start with the Jin Shin Jyutsu treatments everything becomes easier. I gently ask whoever is holding my toes if they would be willing to close their eyes and then share with me what they "see." It turns out that everyone does see something—everyone has a visual metaphor for fighting this cancer. We're surprised to discover how often our imagery matches, but sometimes their energy and enthusiasm leads my inner vision to new places. My most recent image is hopeful.

My lung is full of needles like pins stuck in a pincushion— all of them puncturing the tumor.

Before leaving Connecticut I dance onstage with my niece Sarah's dance troupe. I can't match the flexibility of their 13-year old bodies, but I join their spirits and they lift mine—and the imagery evolves again.

Increasingly the dancers are successful in popping the bubble wrap. The stage becomes a large gymnasium that is rapidly becoming engulfed in rising bubbles.

Nephew Ted is lead saxophone in the Vermont All-State jazz band at the Burlington *Discover Jazz Festival*. The vibrancy of their performance combined with the emotion of the last week opens my inner life further and brings new dancers to the stage.

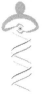

The ballet dancers are joined by break-dancers who spin on their backs and heads to take down as many bubbles as possible in an endless stream of motion. Ballerinas in white glide; male dancers leap; hip-hoppers pound; break-dancers windmill. There is so much activity that I can't see the other side of the room for all the bubbles. Now the dancers are joined

by acrobats carrying giant poles, which they plant in the floor of my lung before vaulting themselves high in the air.

The poles take on a function beyond entertainment when bubbles start spiraling up the poles. This is their emergency exit, a way to rapidly clear the air and evacuate the building in an orderly fashion.

In August, coming back from our second family reunion (this one with Kelly's extended family), I glance at the airport newsstand while we wait for our luggage to arrive. On the cover of *Popular Science* magazine, in bold red type, is the headline "Cancer Cures" and I eagerly leaf through the magazine to read more. The article talks about miniscule molecular robots called nanobots, which someday will be able to precisely target a cancer cell and deliver a deadly payload. Unfortunately they won't arrive in time to help me, but the picture on the next page does. It shows me what the death of a cancer cell looks like: an explosion of cell debris and water that looks just like my bubble meditations (see figure 1). I burst out laughing. How did my visualizations come up with such an accurate picture of a biological process that my conscious mind knows nothing about?

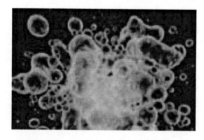

Figure 1. A photograph of the death of a cancer cell in *Popular Science* magazine.

Turning Toward the Light

Next on the healing plan is the sun.

Sun worshipping isn't unusual in the Northwest, where our nearest star hides from us nine months of every year. But most people don't realize that during the other three months it is our constant companion, and in 2006 those three months stretched to five. I lust after the sun. Just turning my head to the light makes me feel better.

Walking is my primary source of solar infusion. The popular trail around Green Lake near Camilla and Isaac's house moves in and out of lightly dappled shade with plenty of open stretches of sunlight. While Kel, Camilla, Isaac, and nephew John play pitch-and-putt golf, Thea and I build up my endurance by walking around the lake. I eagerly put on the sling and carry her extra weight, even adding to my respiratory load by singing or humming to her. Everyone we pass smiles at the beautiful baby in the sling and their good will washes over me too. I exult when I can make the three miles around the lake (earning me Dr. Eaton's "Most Miles Walked" at my next appointment).

Exercise is not the biggest payoff. If Thea falls asleep on my chest, she becomes a transdermal chemo port infusing healing deep into my body and spirit. Her head snuggled into my shoulder is a little furnace of vitality. A bubble of love surrounds us, intimate yet permeable, giving me the sensation of how the body is supposed to work.

Rejoined by the golfers, we head for margaritas for them (Tarceva is taxing my liver enough), a salad for me (I'm eating lots of dark fruits and vegetables, skipping the sugar), and easy laughter for all at the Mexican restaurant near the lake. I make sure I sit in the sunniest chair at the sunniest table. I am phototropic, stretching toward the light, and though the word is defined in terms of plants, you've only got to sit on a Mexican beach in

February surrounded by Northwesterners to know that people, too, seek the light.

When we're on Whidbey I walk almost daily with my friends on the beach, or with Kel at South Whidbey State Park. An old logging road heads into the majestic, magical part of the old-growth forest where shafts of light appear infrequently and unexpectedly. The earth is spongy from centuries of accumulation and the air smells so clean I can't help but inhale deeply. *Breathe this oxygen, it's here for you. Let it nourish your cells and burn out the cancer. Let it cleanse you from deep within.*

This three-mile loop not only exercises my lungs, it strengthens my body with a steep uphill climb to the ridge and the meandering return to the trailhead. In 2008 researchers in England will document the physical and mental health benefits of "green exercise" and in 2010 Harvard will publish those results in its health newsletter.[28] But they will only be stating the obvious to anyone who stands at the feet of these 500-year-old survivors and breathes in.

Back at home my outer world enters my inner world when I listen to *Self-healing With Guided Imagery,* a CD by Dr. Martin Rossman. He invites me to envision a safe healing place.

I start on the same path we walked this morning at the State Park, but it leads to a high, forested trail that opens up into a clearing. I immediately know it is my healing glen. It reminds me of the Ventana Wilderness of California where Kelly and I spent a wondrous afternoon knowing for the first time—without either of us voicing it—that we would spend our lives together.

My inner healer, my goddess, is waiting, and she opens her arms to me. It feels so good to surrender to her embrace, releasing all my tension and worry, basking in her complete love, forgiveness, and compassion.

So this is what prayer must feel like. In the totality of the love, its ease, and its gentleness, I understand my religious friends and relatives better.

At first I rely on one song to transport me quickly to this place but soon I can arrive whenever I need it. I come here when I am full of strength and ready to actively heal, and I come here when I'm depleted and need comfort.

Perhaps I've been drawn to sunlight so much lately because my awareness of shadow remains deep and persistent. However, just as in June the hours of daylight far outnumber the hours of night in the northern skies, light has been prevailing over darkness in my body.

To: My wonderful support team
From: Diana
Date: June 24, 2006
Subject: Diana update

To my wonderful support team,

We are all doing a great job! The CT scan of my lung today showed that the tumor has shrunk to less than ¼ of its original size! And yesterday's MRI of the brain revealed no new tumors there. We are all so excited. My doctor says he'll put my case in the book he plans to write. Thank you so much for your love and support. And when you can manage it please keep doing whatever you're doing, because it's working.

Much love,
Diana

Drafting Energy From Those Who Have It Most

At the end of June when we move back into our house it is no longer a single-family dwelling, it is part of an informal Lindsay

Family Compound. Tom, Susan, John, and Jake now live next door, and a stone path leads from their deck down the gully between our houses and up the hill to the large maple tree by our driveway. Dinner is usually for ten, although it can easily be twenty. Susan bears the brunt of the hospitality and she handles it graciously and generously.

Everyone who gets near me holds my fingers and toes, and initially the strongest energy comes from the younger generation. The twenty-somethings—Camilla, Isaac, Jessie, Seth, and Molly—bring the vitality of new marriages, first steps to parenthood and careers, the surge that comes with their growing sense of competence. The teens—nieces Sabina and Sarah and nephews John, Jake, Calvin, and Ted—bring a raw exuberance, an untamed life force. They all want desperately to give me "the cure" with their hugs, or, if that's beyond their reach, to let me know how much they love me. Perhaps we *are* here to make final memories, but I'd prefer to just enjoy this present moment. I watch how they hang out, how they sprawl over the couches and each other, seemingly in chill mode, yet always with an antennae out for the next moment of spontaneity. If anyone has an idea, they all jump up at once like a flock of birds.

Researchers tell us that mirror neurons are what allow birds to sense each other's intent during migration. In humans, mirror neurons enable us to read faces, emotions, and intentions, to learn vicariously from others and to have empathy for them. These brain cells were first discovered in monkeys when Italian scientists learned that the same part of a monkey's brain fired whether it watched a researcher lift a glass or the monkey itself did so. "We are exquisitely social creatures," says Giacomo Rizzolatti, a neuroscientist at the University of Parma. "Mirror neurons allow us to grasp the minds of others not through conceptual reasoning but through direct simulation. By feeling, not by thinking."[29]

My resonance with these young people makes me wonder whether my mirror neurons could allow me to feel their energy flowing through my body as freely and powerfully as it does through theirs. I follow their spontaneity; they follow my courage. We laugh together. When their mirror neurons enable Isaac and John to feel Kel's pain and anxiety, they take him golfing.

The teens and twenty-somethings share something important with Kelly and me. None of us knows what the hell we are going to do next. At this stage of our lives during the months of June, July, and August, we don't have a schedule. We don't know where we're heading. We don't know how the story's going to unfold—or end. We're just trying as hard as we can to play along the way. We're hoping for an endless summer.

For about 45 minutes before I go to sleep at night and right after I wake up in the morning, I grab headphones from my bedside table, still my mind, and re-enter my inner healing space. It's fun, and it's where I want to be. It's like pressing "Play" on an early VCR machine: I fully expect to return to where we left off but there's always a moment of waiting to see if the machinery of my mind will truly function and the dancers appear. Once I see them, my job is simply to relax, watch, and listen.

The dancers' job, however, is to heal. During any given meditation the scene might not really advance; the action—whether it's pounding, stomping, scrubbing, chipping, or beaming—tends to be repetitive, meticulous, and can last for weeks. The actors—dancer, goddess, water, or light—are careful to leave no harmful cell behind. But the dancers and goddesses also seem as eager to communicate with me as I am with them, doing their best to entertain me with flights of creativity, amusement, and absurdity—anything to keep me in the meditative stillness longer, to delay the time when I press "Pause."

Kel is helping, too. Out of love for me, he has gotten serious about Jin Shin. He has not only devoured a book on it, he's taken the clothes and hair off a Ken doll so he can draw the energy meridians on it with colored pens. His green and yellow flashcards of Jin Shin sequences constantly stick out of his shirt pocket. As he learns to lengthen his treatments, I extend the amount of time my mind stays focused. As he increases his commitment his energy feels stronger to me than that of men twenty years younger.

Whenever my own energy starts to flag or my anxiety rise, Kelly restores my equilibrium. Because I don't have to wait days or weeks for an appointment, a session, or a class before the panic subsides, my body spends less time recovering from fear and more time recovering from cancer. He's so good at steadying me, yet I'm aware of the difficulty his logical mind must be going through trying to wrap itself around something so foreign, and I appreciate just how far this man has been willing to stretch in order to help me.

The Healing Team Is Growing

Living with cancer on Tarceva is not living with cancer in a way that any of us have witnessed in a grandparent, parent, or even in people our own age. Friends who have brought casseroles, driven to chemo appointments, and held bedside vigils for other cancer-stricken friends quickly recognize that I don't need this kind of help. They are a bit incredulous at my Joy Protocol yet look for ways to embrace and expand it. We stroll barefoot in the sand, lie under the stars on blankets at concerts, make books together, and take impulsive road trips. They surround me with only love and kindness.

They even bring the regimen into their own lives. "I took a Diana Day," one of them tells me. "It was just too beautiful not to enjoy."

But what to do the day after that? How do you keep love and joy flowing every day? Eight friends have decided that the answer is a weekly massage and give me eight sessions as a gift. I ask Dr. Eaton if massage is OK.

"We used to think that massage was contra-indicated because we feared that helping the lymph system circulate would spread the cancer, but that's been disproven. There's no study that says it *does* help but if it makes you feel better, go ahead." (Maybe there's no study in 2006 but in 2010 researchers will demonstrate that deep massage significantly decreases the stress hormone cortisol and increases the number of lymphocytes in the immune system.[30] In 2011, researchers will show that massage turns off genes associated with inflammation and turns on genes associated with muscle healing.[31])

The massage therapist, Jill Clark, believes her manipulations will move toxic by-products out of the muscles and into the lymph system for recycling. As she digs in I immediately realize that her two-hour massages provide an opportunity, like with Kel, to have a partner in meditation. So we don't chitchat. As Jill methodically works I return to my body's stage and use the time to replenish all my body's other systems that have been selflessly taking a back seat to the lung.

Jill also offers advice for when I'm off her table. "Your left side is lazy. It's not doing its share and the right side just automatically takes the load. Make a conscious effort to lift things with your left hand and wear Thea on your left hip when you carry her. Stop treating it like the injured party and tell it to step up."

I have found a straight-shooting coach, and I get to spend two hours a week with her. My healing team is growing.

Down the street I find a cheerleader. Dr. Bob Sleight, a chiropractor, takes one look at me and says, "You're going to kick this." He never wavers in his conviction. He believes that chiropractic will help improve my nerve flow, resulting in better communication in my body. Whether he's right or not matters less to me than that he believes in me.

After my various appointments I always feel better. And when I worry that any given pain might be the cancer growing, I don't have to wait through two stressed-out months for my next brain and lung scans to find out. If the pain is gone after seeing Jill or Bob, it's not cancer.

My inner imagery continues to change; now the dancers are no longer the main event and the healing glen is expanding.

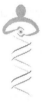 *The goddess leads me to a river adjacent to the glen. She stands on the shore while I enter the water and stand with the sun shining on my face. As I face downstream, the water starts to flow over my shoulders and down my chest like a waterfall. The river brings me all the nutrients my cells need to flourish and carries downstream all the toxins my cells—including the cancer—have expelled. Over time an inner channel forms, entering through my scapula and flowing down inside my body through the spaces between cells, and then out my navel. The goddess and I can stay here indefinitely, warmed by the sun overhead and cooled by the stream flowing through me.*

I repeat this meditation over and over in my head, even when I'm not in a meditative state. I start to believe that it is as important to rid my body of dead cancer cells as it is to kill them in the first place.

The imagery in the healing glen has come from physical places I'd already been, but now my river meditations are also starting to suggest places I could go. It's no longer enough to see the images only in my mind; I need to experience them in person. So Kelly and I start chasing waterfalls. After hiking to Narada Falls at Mt. Rainier, I cry out to Kel: "This is the perfect place! See how the water breaks around that rock as if it's flowing down both shoulders?" But we can't quite get close enough. So we seek out more waterfalls: the large but hidden Spray Falls also at Rainier, two in Vermont, a tiny one by the shore of the Skykomish River in Washington State, and the towering Vernal Falls at Yosemite. Next to each one I repeat the waterfall visualization in my mind as I listen to the roar of the water: good nutrients in, toxins out, in an endless flow.

The hiking itself—the distances, elevation, and clean air pumping through me—is healing, but I have an intuition that there is something more going on here. The saying *As above so below, as within so without* keeps running through my mind as I search for the universal principles of water—the molecules that make up 60% of the human body, 70% of the brain, and 90% of the lungs.[32] If, as an old joke goes, my body is just a container that water invented so it could walk around,[33] then how does that water itself work? What is its optimal condition? How does water purify itself? How does it break through obstructions and overcome stagnation? Perhaps the basic ways that any cell absorbs light, excretes waste, and takes in water would work in my body as well. So I watch, I breathe in the spray, I get into the water wherever I can (or I imagine the power of the falls flowing over me), and I encourage my water cells to be all they can be.

Surfing brain waves

Sometimes it feels like I'm living on three planes simultaneously. I live what I once would have called a normal life, aware of what's going around me and capable of focusing and interacting with anyone. But there's a background hum that rarely leaves me, a steady anxiety that tells me not to get too attached to this world because I am soon going to leave it. The third plane is the inner world of my meditations and imagery. This is the most compelling place for my brain to hang out.

During the waiting period between scans I wonder how much I can trust my internal images to tell me how I'm doing. Are they offering glimpses of what is truly happening in my body, or just what I want to happen? Am I the one signaling an intention to my body to heal, or is my body doing all the communicating to me? Some messages I'm receiving instinctively feel truer, more authentic, than others, as if they come from a deeper source within my body. I find myself more apt to believe a message when the images change spontaneously without my direction, when they surprise me.

I discover a possible explanation for all this at a museum exhibit called "Mindball," in which two people don headsets that monitor their brain wave patterns, face each other, and try to out-relax each other. If you are more relaxed than your partner, your ball moves toward the finish line. But if you open your eyes and get excited about being ahead, you lose ground. (There must be a moral in here somewhere.) When I put the headset on, my family watches my brainwaves on a display monitor. Even in the presence of competing exhibits with bells and videos, I'm so relaxed that I nearly bottom out the display of alpha and theta waves.

It turns out there are four types of brainwaves, each progressively slower. We use:

- *Beta waves* to engage in everyday activity that requires thought and concentration;
- *Alpha waves* to daydream, create, worry, or zone out as we drive on the freeway;
- *Theta waves* to meditate and to dream; they provide a gateway between being awake and asleep that you can access from either state;
- *Delta waves* to provide us with the state of deep sleep without dreaming.

Researchers have found that we use multiple brain wave patterns at the same time. This excites me because it's a possible explanation for why I feel like I'm living on three planes. What if information that felt dictated, invented, focused, or contrived, like my mind telling my body what to do or my mind remembering what my imagery was about, was carried by beta waves? What if information that wasn't particularly informative, like anxiety or relaxation, was brought to me by alpha waves?[34] What if the information that felt closest to the truth was carried by theta waves[35]—which would explain why this language is so visual and dreamlike, why I can access these images more easily coming into and out of sleep, and why it feels like a deeper kind of knowing? I have been looking for a place in my brain that would serve as the portal to my autonomic healing system, but maybe what's required is a new state of being.

There's one other song that plays constantly in my brain these days, and perhaps it's carried by a frequency that researchers are just discovering in Buddhist monks, the gamma wave: it's a song of gratitude to be thinking and breathing at all.

To: My wonderful support team
From: Diana
Date: August 25, 2006
Subject: Diana Update August

Hello wonderful support team,

It's been two months since my last CT scan, which, as you may recall, showed that the tumor was half of what it was the month before, which itself was half of the original tumor. Apparently this cancer is behaving just like two people sharing a pie who keep halving the last bite, because today's CT showed that it halved yet again! By my math, that's 1/8th of the original size, but the doctor said "maybe even less." Apparently math acts differently when you have to take into the account the volume of very strange shapes. We are very excited! And so is my doctor. While looking at the scans he said in a quiet voice, "maybe we can get rid of this"—the first time he has acknowledged that possibility. Of course, that's been our plan all along, so I'm thinking that with your help we should just eat that last bit of pie and clean the plate.

If you have the patience to keep doing what you're doing, thank you! Let's just whup this by Thanksgiving, the approximate time of my next CT.

Love,
Diana

CHAPTER FOUR

Two Steps Forward, One Step Back

August, 2006–July, 2007

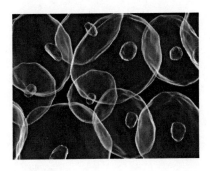

"I can't keep it all going, Diana, I'm so sorry," says Nancy, our business partner, as we talk at the small round table in my office in early August.

With the current state of insurance in this country, I'm in a bind. I have to go back to work to keep it but I'm afraid if I do, I will only get sicker. But this is not Nancy's problem.

"Nancy, you were never under any obligation to keep the company going. You've been incredibly generous these past months and I'm grateful to you for keeping everyone employed for this long," I answer, "but I don't think I can take back the stress of sales. Maybe we have to close the doors."

I'm really not thinking clearly now. This would be a hardship on our staff and on us—and with my cancer as a pre-existing condition, how would I ever get other insurance?

But fortunately Nancy doesn't want Lindsay Communications to end any more than I do. We talk about the load she's been carrying, which parts seem manageable, and which parts push her over the top. "If you could take over the big consulting job, I think I can keep going with the rest," she offers. I'm happy to agree.

This only means working four days in August, but by September I am back at the job in a big way. I try to limit myself to half days, but when crises arise—and they always do—my days stretch to as many as 10 hours. This starts to concern me, and to terrify Kel. It's not that I haven't built back enough strength to handle it, and it's not that the work environment is overly stressful. It's just that I don't believe it's contributing to my health. Now I'm spending too much time in my left brain when I was making real progress exploring the right. Work may be the responsible and financially prudent thing to do but it is taking time away from the healing plan and no longer feels safe for me.

⊙ ⊙ ⊙

In the last few weeks I've experienced some pressure and pain in my chest, so we're relieved when Dr. Eaton tells us that my October 4 scan indicates the tumor has not grown. At that moment we are so happy that neither Kelly nor I register that the tumor has stopped shrinking. We are so happy to not be going backwards that it takes us a while to realize we're also not going forward.

Tarceva was originally approved because it lengthened survival time from 4.7 to 6.7 months. I'm at six months now, so perhaps we've reached the end of this miracle. I've been the one asserting the cancer could go into remission, but that has never been Dr. Eaton's claim. I start waking up in the morning terrified, upset, and vulnerable. It doesn't help that I'm losing half my hair. It takes a few hours to talk myself into feeling good again, and it's a struggle the rest of the day to hang on to that frame of mind.

Kel and I become consumed with trying to figure out what I've been doing differently, but for all our theories we have no way of knowing why the cancer has stopped shrinking. Work is an obvious scapegoat, but that only started up recently. To compound the dilemma, Kel starts to blame himself: was he slacking on the Jin Shin Jyutsu treatments? My brain strains to figure out what it is that helps me heal and what doesn't, but maybe I'm not the one in control here; the cancer might have its own sense of direction, or timing. Doesn't common wisdom tell us that the last inch/mile/pound/bit of tumor is always the hardest to lose?

Instead of imagining all the car crashes that could lie ahead, I steady myself by looking at the intersection I'm driving through today: with the tumor at roughly 2 centimeters by 1 centimeter, I'm still in pretty good shape. I'm strong, I have lung power, and I can hike up hills more easily than I have for years. I've lost half my hair but I have a drawer full of new headbands. And I have a new idea.

"Nancy, I think I can train Monica to take over my role. If I finish this strategic consulting job by December, would you be willing to keep things going while I mentor Monica?"

Again, Nancy says yes.

I go home and start to write down everything I've learned in twenty years of business. It's a gift to be able to pass it on to another. "Monica, this will have to be a six-month course, since I'm supposed to be dead by April. I sincerely hope that won't be the case, but you should be ready to take over by then."

The Gratitude Tour

Prepare for the worst in life as in business. The *LiveStrong Survivorship Notebook* that Kel's cousin has just sent calls this "Practical Topics." Living will. Power of attorney. Estate planning. Getting your affairs in order. We've taken stabs at these before. When we procrastinated, our attorney Doug put handwritten post-its on the legal documents: "While I know you're busy, I also know you're mortal." We used to think these notes were humorous.

Kelly takes care of the legal documents because I have little interest in them. When I contemplate the accounting of a lifetime I don't think of money, I think of relationships. For the past months, I've been trying to reach by email everyone who has graced my life since I was five. Now, knowing we're going to Northern California for four days to hear our son Eric's latest composition performed, I am driven to reconnect in person. I fill my calendar with promises to see friends, colleagues, students and mentors from the two decades Kel and I spent there.

In California we meet in the morning light at a kitchen table, or the midday light at a local cafe, or the waning light in a wine bar. We gather in constellations that haven't been aligned for thirty years and we talk long into the night. Our conversations fill in the missing DNA strands of our lives, clear up youthful misperceptions, and reveal the impact we've had in each other's lives.

I don't ask anything of anyone; after months of receiving I want to be the giver, to thank them, to be sure they know how much I love them. Of course it doesn't work out quite that way. They remind me that I have had strength, resilience, and a willingness to buck the system for a long time. And when we unlock the memory of two first graders in love with the same boy, I can see the petticoat dresses, hear the laughter on the playground, and feel the chemistry of a friendship that has lasted 48 years. While I take note of the competent executive in front of me, I remember his preppy haircut, hear the flute in the resonant dorm stairwell, and feel the excitement of that first night of college. When I hug colleagues and students from my first job, I put to rest the insecurities I felt at the time and am grateful for all they taught me about the joys of creative collaboration. The chemicals might have lost some of their original potency since my brain stored them, but they are still there, and as I reopen the memory drawers I release their healing power.

Gratitude is its own reward, too, a serenity that reminds me that the richness in my life is already enough. And of course, practically speaking, I have just done a very effective job of recruiting more wonderful people to my healing team, for whatever comes next.

The hands of the goddess are working on the lymph nodes between my lungs. Over and over, she massages them with a strong pressure.

I don't know whether the goddess is so intent on these lymph nodes because of new growth there, or because she's removing the existing cancer, but it's interesting to note that the current recommended medical treatment for lymphedema, the swelling of the lymph nodes, is massage.

⊙⊙⊙

After decades of business travel I've come to the conclusion that a plane is an over-stuffed can of viruses and bacteria. My luggage may or may not have shifted in the overhead compartment during flight, but my sinuses consistently succumb to invaders. But somehow I had forgotten the risk I was taking by flying to Europe during flu season to teach back-to-back business training sessions in two different countries.

By noon the first day the virus I met on the plane has hijacked my larynx. After the first training I take a long befuddled taxi ride back to my hotel in Madrid—leaving my purse in the cab—and crawl into bed where I stay until our train leaves for Paris. It's hard to feel sorry for a visitor to Paris, but if anyone qualifies right now it would be me. At 4:00 a.m., with my sinuses locked up and a hacking cough, I panic. I am afraid that my cancer is resurgent, and I am a long way from Dr. Eaton. Kelly and I call our son Eric and ask him to arrange for someone else to teach the next class for me. Kel calls the airline to get us on the next plane back home.

This time I am the one filling the air ducts with nasty germs. The poor man next to me seems tolerant as I cram one used tissue after another into the airsick bag, but I'm sure inwardly he's kissing his upcoming work week goodbye. Kel and I have an appointment to see Dr. Eaton the next day.

"You did the right thing," he says. "Pneumonia in a lung cancer patient is not a pretty thing." Nor, it turns out, is my next scan.

The radiologist notes an "ill-defined opacity" in my left lung, *probably* the result of pneumonia. Or is it the cancer taking up a new outpost? This is the beginning of my education in the art—as opposed to the science—of CT scans. Radiologists are required to note everything they see in their reports, but what they see is not necessarily significant. Nor does cancer always announce itself with neon lights. It turns out that there are gray areas—ill-defined opacities—in both medicine and life.

However, there's also good news. The cancer in my lymph nodes is gone, "resolved" in radiology parlance. The timing of the goddess massage meditation on November 22 is so close to my December clinical results that I start to wonder whether the visualizations could possibly be reflecting my body's status even before the CT verifies it.

The Dance Changes

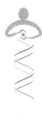

As the tumor shrinks the dancers try to fit onto an increasingly smaller space. Their movement has changed as a result; they are like Balkan dancers now, jumping straight up and down on narrow mountaintops because they don't have enough real estate for larger movement. Unfortunately their stomping is not working, because instead of the easily destroyed bubble surface they danced on before, they now dance on a hard, small, lava-like spire. It is difficult work, and they are not successful.

The presence of the "ill-defined opacity" and the sense that the dancers aren't getting anywhere amplifies my anxiety about my upcoming scan. Kel can see when I wake up this morning that my night has been full of bad dreams, and my stress level threatens to make the day no better.

He brings me to the couch for a Jin Shin treatment, and we review our strategies for coping with fear over these last nine months.

1. *The boat.* I imagine that fear is a toy sailboat that I see, recognize, and acknowledge but let float down the stream without giving it any more energy. I find out later that this is a mindfulness meditation technique for quieting the brain, but given that I have no training in mindfulness meditation, you can imagine how successful this is.

2. *The "don't waste my time."* Here I think that if the very worst happens, I will never be healthier or happier than I am today, so why waste a moment of today worrying about something that may never happen? This requires the presence of logic and therefore only works if anxiety is low.

3. *The "I think I can and dammit I will."* When I'm playing with Thea I get so angry at the thought that I won't get to spend a lifetime with her that I strengthen my resolve to will this sucker away. This actually works for a while, one medium-burn emotion being replaced by another that's more consuming.

4. *Deep breaths.* Sometimes the anxiety stays with me and I take deep breaths to release it, or I use a technique from Dr. Weil's *Breathing*[36] audiotape: inhale for a count of 4, hold the breath for a count of 7, and slowly release it for a count of 8. This works. The breath unlocks the knot in my solar plexus where the anxiety lives.

5. *Visualization.* My inner goddess puts her arms around me in the healing glen and holds me. I feel loved and the anxiety dissolves, freeing me to actively work with my inner healers. This works the best.

Now that we've begun talking about this, we remember a sixth strategy—*distraction*. When my life is full, I forget to be afraid. Which is why we realize the best responses to fear are also the best tools for healing: love, music, touch, and exercise. We leave our list behind as we head to the State Park.

⊙ ⊙ ⊙

My January 26, 2007 CT shows the size of the tumor has stabilized. It looks like the earlier shrinkage was a bonus, and this mass is the size we will have to live with. But there is something to celebrate: the ill-defined opacity is gone, along with all symptoms of the pneumonia. So I agree to take on a new intense project at work in early February. And by the end of that month something new shows up in my imagery.

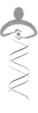

The healer is swimming around between cells and comes across a large one that doesn't look like either the nice little bubble wrap that the dancers have been smashing, or the lava-like spires that have been more stubborn. This cell is different. Its outside perimeter has tentacles like the roots of a tree. The goddess wants to carve around the cell to extract it, like she did with the brain lesions before Gamma Knife, but she can't see its borders clearly. She is afraid that if she cuts too closely, she will leave behind some roots.

Then she comes up with a solution. She thinks of the cell as a rubber glove. If she fills it with fluid, the glove itself will identify its boundaries. So she takes a syringe and fills the cell with a pink liquid. The cell quickly inflates, and she turns it inside out and stands it on end, like an upright tree. She then zaps it with a giant burst of light, and it is gone.

The moment this meditation is over I know it's significant, and I connect it to an article I'd read several days earlier by surgeon Diane Simeone, director of gastrointestinal oncology at the University of Michigan Comprehensive Cancer Center:

> "Doctors have long wondered what makes some cancers so hard to treat. While some tumors wither under radiation or chemotherapy, or are easily cut away with surgery, others grow back, sometimes years later, despite even the harshest therapies. These relapses often prove fatal, taking the lives of patients who appeared cancer free.
> New research suggests that a small group of especially hardy cells may be to blame. Doctors call them cancer stem cells.
>
> Although few in number—they make up less than 1% of a tumor—cancer stem cells may be the driving force behind many tumors, playing a far more central and lethal role than the more numerous and ordinary cancer cells that surround them."[37]

The tree-glove is a stem cell, I conjecture, and I have to tell someone about it. Scientists have been discovering stem cells for different cancer types, but as of April 2006 they have not yet found the stem cell for lung cancer. The dream makes me start to question therapies, like Tarceva, that only target the outside perimeter of the cell. I believe it's significant that the cell will reveal its own nature if you can somehow get into its center.

I've been getting headaches, so I call Dr. Eaton to move up my bi-monthly brain MRI; I don't want to spend a month worrying about whether a new tumor has emerged. Afterwards, he calls to let me know the preliminary radiologist report says there's nothing there.

"Never have I been so grateful for the common headache," I reply.

"Enjoy," he responds.

Later in the day he calls back. "Not only is there nothing to worry about; all the brain lesions and even the scarring from the Gamma Knife are gone."

I've been so focused on a worst-case scenario that it takes a while for this additional news to register. I even call the nurse to reread the report to be sure I've heard correctly. The only downside is that if I lose my keys, I can no longer blame it on brain cancer.

To: Love-In attendees
From: Diana
Date: April 8, 2007
Subject: You're invited to the Love Back Party April 21st 6 pm

It's almost been a year since I was diagnosed and you all gathered me and mine in your arms at the Love-In. I am now 55, still alive, and wanting to thank you for all the love and support you have given us over this year. So we're having a Love Back party on April 21st at 6:00. You and your family and anyone else hanging around your house are welcome.

You were all so good at following the rules of the Love-in (my sock drawer still thanks you) that I thought I'd try again with the rules of the Love Back: There are no rules for Love Back parties. Love is limitless. The rules come before the party: don't bring anything. There is one exception: If you're a fellow cancer survivor and you'd like to thank this community too then bring a token something to eat or drink to put you on the giving side of things.

Thank you from the bottom of our hearts and we hope to see you soon,
Diana and Kelly

Now each day with Thea is part of a succession of milestones: first stair-climb; first "no"; first gallop; first solo; first singing together. Our children, too, are piling up dates on the calendar that beckon me forward like signs on a highway. See Isaac's opening in Seattle in February. Be in New York in May to watch Eric accept a Young

Composer Award at Lincoln Center. Watch Kylie cross the stage to get her PhD from UCLA in June. We celebrate what our children have accomplished and the fact that I'm still here to see it.

Then Camilla throws me another life preserver. She is pregnant again. I can barely breathe when I think that I might not make it to our second grandchild's birth, and I'm fiercely determined to make it happen. Friends also invite me to share their milestones, keeping me moving in life's swift current: sing at my wedding; knit with me while I wait for my first labor to begin; share my grief at the death of my mother. They all keep me off the couch and on the road. When I first sat down to write my bucket list I wanted to be with family more than travel to exotic destinations, but now I seem to be doing both.

When I tell Dr. Eaton about our latest wanderings, he gives me a gold star for "Doing the Most with the Time Given." What is that if not a life?

My definition of a milestone is also changing. I'm not less appreciative of the big moments, I'm just more appreciative of the small ones. I used to wrap myself in the illusion of my immortality like bulletproof glass, but now that it's shattered I feel vulnerable and exposed—not so much to death as to life. Colors are richer, sounds more vibrant, time more elastic. I can smell my oxygen exchange with the old-growth trees in our forests and feel both the pleasure and the calm of walking them with old-growth friends. I can taste adrenaline, and I no longer want its metallic flavor dominating others in my life. I can feel love as both a chemical and energetic exchange. Nature has hidden medicine everywhere, and joy is helping me absorb it.

But it is not only joy that I come to appreciate as I near my 16-month milestone. I appreciate the trauma in my life for the resilience it has taught me and the cancer for how it has woken me up. I call it my "And" life. The evil *and* the good. The euphoria *and* the pain. It has all lead me to this moment of truly being happy. It also includes a return to my previous life and my roles as grandmother, parent, and consultant. I try to do what's needed in as stress-free a way as possible, although I don't always succeed.

Kel and I spend the summer canoeing. When the river flows slowly, there's time to put our paddles down and appreciate the flight of a heron. When the current tugs more urgently, our focus narrows to the strength of our strokes and the distance to the bank. But we're most alert and engaged when we hear the roar of the rapids before we see them, and have only seconds to decide our course. It is good training. We are about to go over the falls.

CHAPTER FIVE

Radiating the Body, Enlightening the Mind

August–December, 2007

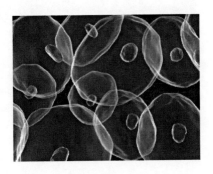

My performance levels have been so good that Dr. Eaton has extended the intervals between my lung and brain scans. Now that it's been four months, it's time for another look.

No matter how good you feel, waiting for scan results is excruciating, so our friends Rene and Miles have volunteered to distract us by taking us to the mountains and cooling us off in Icicle Creek. Without naming it, the four of us conduct our own test of my health: Can I hike seven miles at Mile's active pace and still laugh at dinner?

I feel so exhilarated and alive that I'm certain that the scans will show the cancer retreating. Looking at myself in the cabin mirror as I brush my teeth, I want to write Love, Joy, and Determination on the mirror with lipstick. I think that if having cancer has led to my feeling this euphoric, then bring it on. Full of confidence, I invite Rene and Miles to witness cancer in retreat at my follow-up appointment on the way back home.

Some retreat.

We are shocked when Dr. Eaton tells us that the chest CT shows the Tarceva starting to lose effectiveness, and the presence of a new tumor that is already 1 cm across.

Dr. Eaton doesn't look overjoyed either.

"Unfortunately the clinical trial I told you about earlier has closed and a new one is maybe two months out. So I think we should try chemotherapy."

"But how long would that give me?" I ask, knowing that chemotherapy isn't effective against stage IV lung cancer.

"Two to four months," he answers. Of a poor quality of life, I add to myself.

"What about CyberKnife?" I blurt out.

"Why? Have you heard the ads for it on the radio?" he responds.

No, that's not it. I've been keeping a folder labeled *Alternative Treatments*, which could also be called the *When-All-Goes-South* file. I have cut and pasted every press release from the Cancer Care of America newsletter that pertains to any lung cancer treatment, whether in stage I trials or beyond. The file now contains more than 70 pages. How do I remember CyberKnife, another tightly-targeted radiation therapy, at this particular moment—especially when my brain is not otherwise functioning? I think it's because February's meditation already showed me radiation blasting the stem cells. This fortuitous recall is a gift from my subconscious. In his book *Blink*, Malcolm Gladwell writes that mountains of data and excessive detail can actually do us a disservice, overwhelming our ability to make decisions, yet our intuition can cut through this complexity to find the "thin slice" that is most reflective of what's essential. "And the truth is that our unconscious is really good at this, to the point where thin-slicing often delivers a better answer than more deliberate and exhaustive ways of thinking."[38]

But Dr. Eaton doesn't see it this way at first. He just thinks it's a bad idea: the horse is out of the barn, we can't have a targeted treatment when it's a systemic problem, etc., etc.

Kel and I go home, struggling to make sense of it, but end up just going to sleep in hopes that tomorrow will bring some direction. But the shoulder ache that yesterday I would have attributed to canoeing, or carrying Thea, now feels more like cancer pain.

To: Wonderful Support team
From: Diana
Date: September 12, 2007
Re: Bad, better, best

Hello my wonderful support team,

The bad part

My CT on Aug. 20 showed a new tumor, which probably

indicates that Tarceva is losing effectiveness. We were stunned. The doctor's suggestion of traditional chemo seemed like a slide from a very high quality of life to a very low one. I asked if I would be eligible for a space-age technology called CyberKnife radiation and my doctor said no.

The better part

I woke up the next day with all the fire and clarity that I now know comes after I hear I have a new tumor (having been through this now 4 times). The message was that if I have to keep fighting a deadly force, I need to have a single focus and we need to take care of all the loose ends and "the shit you don't get to." In one day we asked Monica and Linda to take over all daily management of the company (and they heroically accepted; we will remain in an oversight role), extracted Kelly from his part of the work, filmed a fund-raising appeal for the Whidbey Island Center for the Arts, and scheduled meetings with our lawyer and financial planner. Stuff that would normally take us about 10 years to do. Then we set out on Friday the 24th to celebrate our 33rd wedding anniversary, canoe and tandem bike on the roof. On the way to the river the doctor calls to say he has re-thought his strategy, consulted with his partner to make sure he wasn't crazy, and thinks my case is "so out of the box" that CyberKnife could be an option.

The best part

The river was exciting! We paddled down 8 miles with obstacles at every bend, capsized twice, and biked back 6 miles. Nothing like being on the edge to know you're alive. And when we met with one of the pioneers of stereotactic radiation, Dr. Vivek Mehta, he thought I was a "fascinating case." He said that if I had I walked in his office when I was first diagnosed he would have given me 4–6 months to live, and here I am at 16+ months radiantly healthy. He said that either the biology of my cancer was unique, I was unique, or what we were doing was unique, but in any case, no doctor could make a prediction about me without factoring *me* in.

He went on to say that since the cancer has not metastasized in the 16 months since the initial brain lesions were zapped— that "it would be reasonable" to treat me as if I just walked in today—as a stage 2 patient! This opens the door to surgery, or chemo/radiation, or CyberKnife. We decided to honor this body that has performed so well by going with the procedure that will do it the least harm. That's CyberKnife. It will deliver highly targeted radiation to what is now a very small tumor area using 4D imaging and robotics (similar to the Gamma Knife radiation that was so successful on my brain minus the headgear) with hopefully minimal side effects. I have a 70–80% chance of having all the "PET-active," or visible, cancer gone! This is the first time since my diagnosis that odds have been stacked in my favor. This will not mean that I am permanently out of the woods, but 16 months with no symptoms is a pretty great record, and CyberKnife could buy me time while more cancer management drugs come on stream.

We left both offices so elated, so grateful to Tarceva, and so affirmed that what we have all done (and this includes you!) has made such a difference.

Please blast me and the family with love these next two weeks (send some to the insurance company too, so they don't think that out of the box means out of pocket) and let's get rid of this before they lay me on the table! And please send me a list of your Top Ten pieces of music. During the CyberKnife treatment, I've got to lie there and meditate for four hours and I could use some help.

Love,
Diana

To: Diana
From: Targe

We certainly will keep sending joyous energy north to you. You may notice a spike, then a sustained surge, on Tuesday when we return to school and spend seven hours a day with 500+ little living generators.

love, Targe and Barb

Targe,

Why don't you have the kids touch your Love-In bracelet, and then mine will be the receiver?

Love, Diana

Diana,

Just so you know, 366 kids (18 classes of kids) touched my wrist, hand, or bracelet yesterday on the first day of school. About the same number did so again today.

love, Targe

Targe,

On the way home tonight from the PET scan I was recognizing that I had two very different emotions going on simultaneously. One that I was scared and two that I was such a loved and lucky woman. Now I know about the love part.

Thank you so much and thank all of the kids. Wow.

Love, Diana

Puncturing the Status Quo

"Name? Date of birth? Which side are we doing the procedure on?"

A perky nurse rolls her computer over to the bedside to ask a battery of questions before surgery to implant the little, gold BB-like markers in my lung that CyberKnife needs to track my breathing. It's a new computer system and it takes a while. She leaves me lying in the middle of a large room with all the others patients awaiting surgery.

Kelly also has been getting me ready with continuous treatment last night and before heading into the hospital this morning. Our love for each other is my lifeline, and I don't want him to ever let go.

Even with controlled chaos all around me, I am pulled into a deep meditation.

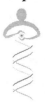

I am back with the goddesses in our healing glen, but the image is shifting. We are moving from the glen to an adjacent meadow. There is a stillness here, a sense of expectation in the shadows of the pine trees that encircle us. We are not alone; my family and friends are coming.

> *They emerge from the woods unbidden, like ballplayers
> coming out of the corn in Field of Dreams. A strong circle
> of silent support, they hold hands around the edges of
> the meadow.*

"Name? Date of birth? Which side are we doing the procedure on?"

Different nurse, same questions. I'm wearing a wristband with my name and birthdate; I have an X already inked on my chest; the medical record is still on the computer screen by my bedside. Though heavily publicized, wrong-site surgeries turn out to be extremely rare.[39] I'm grateful anyway for the nurse's vigilance, but the meadow is far more compelling than repetitive questions I barely answer.

> *The circle is getting bigger. Family and friends on Whidbey
> have now been joined by people from my teens, twenties, and
> thirties. I also recognize my mother's friends—my honorary
> aunts from '50s suburbia.*

> *The circle somehow accommodates each newcomer without
> breaking hands, and starts to gently sway before moving
> clockwise. I step into the center and start spinning, head
> back and arms outstretched, just like I did on my first visit
> to the actual meadow in 1974, when Kel and I got engaged.
> I think to myself: How can I not get well when I have such
> a force behind me?*

"Name? Date of birth? Which side are we doing the procedure on?"

This is Albert, a nurse wearing a red bandana on his head and sporting some attitude. But he takes one look at me, softens, and says, "Wow. I can see that you are really prepared for this. What are you doing?"

When I tell him I'm meditating, he says I won't need much in the way of anesthesia because my tools are better than his.

We roll into pre-op, where I immediately feel that the energy isn't right. The doctor is rushed. It's already 12:30 and he probably hasn't had a chance to eat. He gets my name wrong, thinking Lindsay is my first name. This flusters him; he wishes he had gotten it right. He explains the procedure: "Your surgery will be difficult. I have to plant the markers in a very small spot. I'm going to tell you to hold your breath, and if you don't do exactly as I say I will stick you."

I draw a calming breath, trying to include him in the non-verbal message. Slow down. Relax.

"I will be your best patient," I reassure him. "I have good body control. I will do exactly as you say."

I used to practice dances over and over again with my students, but here—when my lung is on the line—we don't practice even once. Albert gives me a mild dose of sedative so I can stay conscious to work with the surgeon, and in we roll. The screen shows a real-time CT so the surgeon can see my lung expand and contract with every breath. In the diagnostic CT machines I'm familiar with a voice says: "Inhale… Now hold your breath… Breathe." Following that rhythm might have helped us, too, but instead the surgeon just barks: Hold your breath.

I comply but he gives me no cues on when to breathe again. We're OK on the first implant, and perhaps the second one, but on the third I call out: "Albert, something's wrong."

I'm instantaneously back in the meadow. The silent sway of the dance has given way to relaxed banter. People are hugging me. I am happy and safe.

'Diana! Diana!'

> *Hi, old friend, it's so wonderful to see you! Thank you
> for coming.*
>
> *'Diana! Diana!'*

I wake up to a roomful of critical-response doctors and nurses. I've had a vasovagal episode: I've fainted. Or was it code blue? From the waiting room, Kelly watched helplessly as the medical teams rushed into the operating room.

I smile at them. "Well, I'm sorry I caused you some alarm but you didn't need to worry, I was just fine." And I do feel fine, like I've been away in a beautiful place.

As Albert rolls me out, he whispers conspiratorially, "I love your smile. You did great. He says he nicked your bone but actually he punctured your lung. You've got a pneumothorax. We'll monitor you all afternoon and see if it resolves by itself."

Five p.m. is a scary time in hospitals because the staff goes off shift and a decision needs to be made. Admit me, or let me go. It's easier to let me go. I'm strong; I'm smiling. I don't fit the profile of someone with a punctured lung. But that changes several days later when I try to climb quickly up a steep hill after a hilarious dinner with old friends and piercing pain threatens to cut the evening short.

The next morning I call Swedish Hospital. Come right in, they say. But there is no "right in" from Whidbey Island. We drive to the ferry, wait for the ferry, ride the ferry, and get stuck in traffic driving to Seattle. It's 2:30 p.m. before we finally arrive, and it's close to two hours later before I'm sitting in an empty room with two surgeons—the same surgeon who implanted the gold markers and a new one who looks like he's now in charge. Once again we are approaching the 5:00 p.m. witching hour.

"You still have a pneumothorax, and we need to operate

right now to put in a chest tube to drain the air that has built up. Your surgeon is going off duty so I will be doing the surgery. Do you have any questions?" asks the new doctor.

"Can I get my husband?"

They start escorting me to the waiting room in little baby steps. I want none of it and stride out to find Kelly. Behind me I hear one doctor say to the other, "She's the one with the pneumothorax and she's leaving us behind."

Kel quickly goes with the new surgeon to review the X-ray. My original surgeon hangs back.

"I remember you. I've never seen anyone come out of a vasovagal with such calm and peace. I can only hope that if it happened to me I'd be able to do the same."

It is as close to an apology as I will get, and I accept it.

I'm escorted across the hall and told to get up on the operating table. That's it. No gown. No anesthesia. ("Is that okay?" the doctor asks. "The shift is changing and that way we won't have to admit you. Just hold onto this bar. Sure, keep your shoes on if you'd like.") And as the surgeon scrubs his hands and my back, I return to the meadow…

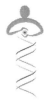

The goddesses are waiting in the healing glen when I enter. Now dressed in work clothes—boots and jeans— they're sitting in the grass and leaning their backs against the marble table.

'Are you ready to do this again?' I ask.

'Of course,' they answer, as they stand up and form a circle, 'but this time, let's put the doctor in the center.' They all laugh as if it's a big joke.

Brilliant! And that's what we do.

I love my goddesses.

They help me for the bulk of the procedure, but even they can't keep me from the searing spike of pain when the surgeon punctures the pleura, the thin membrane that protects and cushions the lungs.

"I didn't tell you about that to keep you from worrying," he says afterward.

The medical team discharges me with thorough instructions but inadequate pain control. When we get to Camilla and Isaac's, I call my friend, Rene, and ask her to send out a phone chain to help me with the pain. Too late. I throw up and pass out in Kel's lap. He starts to yell for help just as I revive, wondering who puked on my robe.

Awake, I find myself in my own nightmare. The nurse we call suggests supplementing the Vicodin with ibuprofen on a two-hour rotating schedule. But even that is not enough and Kelly starts nonstop Jin Shin to help me manage pain that feels like labor without the breaks between contractions. When he presses down strongly on my back I can manage, but somewhere in the night he falls asleep, and I am alone. The pain is more than I can bear, so I look for help.

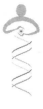 *I rise above a layer of clouds like the swirl of communications encircling the earth in an AT&T commercial. There's Rene. Will you walk with me? She takes my arm, but after a few minutes I let her go, not wanting to overtax her. There's Bonnie, and she strolls with me for a while. Did anyone call Kären? I can see across the clouds to her house. I knock on her door and ask if she, too, will walk with me. I will always walk with you, she replies.*

And so, friend by friend they accompany me through the night until 5:00 a.m., when I wake Kelly to take me to the emergency room. (The pain is so all-consuming that it never occurred to me that emergency rooms are 24/7.) I'm admitted to the hospital for a weekend of morphine while the pneumothorax resolves.

A Visit to the Shaman

One of the difficulties of knowing whether a 1% solution is worth trying is approaching it with a 50% mind. But this is the mind I've brought with me to this round kitchen table in a conventional suburban house complete with white shag rug, wife, and kids. Kelly and I are here at the home of the Native American shaman recommended by a friend. Arranging this meeting has taken longer to schedule than CyberKnife. The shaman himself has undergone a purification ritual for three days, the generosity of which astounds me.

The shaman doesn't fit the mold I've concocted from Hollywood movies. His style is not quiet, calm, elderly, or obviously wise. In fact, he's brash, confrontational, and young. He wastes no energy on a compassionate bedside manner, nor on social graces. He's more like a martial arts instructor, which turns out to be his day job.

"I don't cure cancer," are his first words to me. Okay, that's honest, but then why am I here?

"Cancer is a disease of healers," is his next statement. My mind immediately starts cycling through all the reasons I believe he's wrong.

"You must be a doctor or a nurse," he says confidently.

"No."

"Therapist or social worker."

"No."

"Teacher."

"Well, I used to be, but not any more."

Like I'm completely missing the point, he raises his voice. "Are you the one that everyone comes to with their problems, expecting you to find a solution?"

Bingo. I've even made a business out of it. He nods curtly in response.

It's rainy, but we go outside to a blazing fire, where he burns the tobacco leaves I have been told to bring, fanning the smoke towards me with eagle feathers. I can't relinquish my associations between tobacco and lung cancer enough to find this beneficial.

He tells me he senses grief in me and asks me about my childhood. He is right that my teen years contained deep grief, but doesn't everyone have grief somewhere? Haven't I already dealt with it? Is he really reading my current spirit?

I walk in circles under a blue plastic tarp and stand before him while he assesses my chakras with a crystal that swings from side to side. It suddenly stops in mid-air in front of my heart. I look at him incredulously.

"Put your hand on mine. You'll see that I'm not doing anything to make the crystal move or stop."

And he's right. His hand is not moving as the crystal moves back and forth, until once again it stops at my heart.

Oh, for Pete's sake, I realize with exasperation, the crystal is right. My heart has not been into this since I arrived. I've been acting like a rebellious teen-ager. I rise to the challenge. Words have not been serving us well so far but this is supposed to be about energy, so I shut up, close my eyes, fill my heart with love, and simply let it shine out.

And the crystal moves.

But the shaman is not finished with his tough love approach. "You need a purpose. You need a will to live," he challenges me.

"But I have a will to live."

"What is it?"

"My granddaughter, Thea...."

"Not enough," he interrupts. "All grandparents love their grandchildren, and they still die. You need a purpose of your own. What is it?"

He gives me no time to think. Like a deer caught in the headlights, I blurt out, "Bringing joy to other's lives."

"Do you know how to do that?" It's a real question.

"Yes, I do," it dawns on me.

"How?"

"Well, I've done it all my life." It's true. But in that moment, I don't mention the sing-a-longs, the dancing, the highs of performances, nor the misty-eyed parents who watched them. I answer surprisingly: "Lately people are joyful simply being with me."

This time his nod is one of satisfaction.

"Can you get an eagle feather?"

Thinking of the bald eagles that perch on the tree in front of our house, I say yes.

"Then go get your medicine paddle." The medicine paddle came from a medicine man of the Tlingit tribe in Alaska. It was given to a friend of mine in an hour of need, and he has passed it on to me. I knew I didn't have the training to unlock its power, and the shaman didn't seem to have much interest when he dismissively left it on his kitchen table. Now I run back to retrieve it.

Back by the fire, we proceed. I'm silent and receptive as he chants. To my amazement, he takes the half of an eagle feather that is still tied to the paddle after all of its journeys, cuts it free, and puts its tip into the flames. He holds it as it burns, and fans the smoke upward.

"The eagle will carry your cancer away."

We go inside, where the shaman falls into the dining room

table chair, slaps the paddle on the table, and says, "I have a good feeling about this. Maybe your doctors will be bright enough. Find another eagle feather that is better than the one that was on the paddle and replace it."

The next day, Dr. Mehta scans me again in order to begin the CyberKnife planning process. I confess I was hoping the mass would be gone, but the CT shows there is still plenty for Dr. Mehta to work with. We hope he is brilliant enough to do his work well.

⊙ ⊙ ⊙

My lungs have not fully recovered from the lung puncture. I still can't take a full breath. With only three days to go before CyberKnife, I reach the hospital doctor on call to see if I should be worried.

"Yes, it would be better if your lungs were clear before the radiation."

"Is there anything I can do about it?" I ask. He takes a minute to consider this question.

"Can you get off the couch and walk to the refrigerator?"

"Not a problem."

"Then listen to your body and walk as much as you can without wearing yourself out."

The weekend weather forecast is for blustery rain on Whidbey, so Kelly and I pile in the Prius, punch in *weather.com* on Kel's BlackBerry, and start driving to find sunshine. It looks like our best chance is Walla Walla, in the far southeast corner of Washington State—some six hours away. Long before that, when we reach the other side of the Cascade Mountain Range, we see a shaft of sunlight pierce the cloud cover, so we get out and walk in its limited circle until it disappears.

After hopping from one sun pool to another, we're no further than Yakima and ready for bed. The Yakima State Fair is in full bloom so there's no room in the inn. Or in any of the hotels, motels, or B&Bs in the surrounding area. Finally I call the Cherrywood B&B, some 20 miles away, whose owner, Pepper, says, "I don't have a room, but I've got a tipi." How cool is that? First a shaman, now a tipi. Admittedly it's a fully decked-out, four-poster-bed, plushy-bathrobe kind of tipi, and I don't know if the day's dose of sunshine is being negated by smoke from the campfire, but the night view of stars blanketing the Yakima Valley certainly fills my soul.

In the morning, Pepper suggests that Kel and I walk to Silver Lake. We follow her directions, and after a while I start looking for, well, a lake. Kel's search object is a quaint community nestled in the orchards, so we both walk right past the vineyard called Silver Lake, get lost, and end up hiking eight miles instead of one. But along the way we glimpse another way of life: apple harvesting; the sweet smell of pears; the vineyards for making local wine. And the gunky feeling in my chest is almost gone.

As we drive back over the mountain pass, I know I wouldn't have been feeling this good had we stayed home in the oppressive gray and gloom. The sun would not have come to us. As a friend once told me: If you can't get there from here, you can always get to somewhere you can get there from.

To: Wonderful support team
From: Diana
Date: October 11, 2007
Subject: Amazing

Hello wonderful family and friends,

This has been a life-changing three days. If it works it will be life-changing because I get my life back. If it doesn't, it will still be life-changing. Thank you all for being a part of it because—trust me—you were all there. The short news for those with a long inbox to get through is that the technology is awesome and my only physical symptom is some fatigue. Your love and support was palpable. With the help of the music you suggested, I spent the four hours in my inner meadow convinced that you really had joined me in an epic party that was part Love-In and part Olympic closing ceremony.

For those with more time, here are the questions I wish I could answer for you personally but don't yet have the energy to do.

What's CyberKnife like? (Bonnie's question)

Physically, not much happened at the mega level of my body so hopefully everything happened at the level of the targeted cells. I had an amazingly kind radiation technician, a cancer survivor himself. He exuded warmth and confidence and told me that when he met me he knew I was a survivor because of the powerful energy I have around me (that's actually you, but more on that later). He escorts me into the room (which in addition to Linor, the CyberKnife machine, has lamps, tables, and other items designed to feel like home—think birth center with a linear accelerator in the middle), with me trailing the power cord to my Bose speaker and iPod. He helps me put on my magic LED vest, helps me onto the table and into my custom foam pad, adjusts the iPod volume, wraps me in a warm blanket, and makes sure I'm comfortable. It feels like there should be chocolates on my pillow, he is so caring and the room so cozy.

Then for ninety minutes I don't move, other than to breathe and occasionally swallow. At first I wonder if I'm breathing too deeply? Too shallowly? Too irregularly? Am I swallowing at the right time? But the technician tells me that Linor won't "shoot" if anything is out of tolerance, so I relax into the moment and head for the meadow. During the session I physically feel nothing. Nothing. At the end I get off the table and walk out of the room into my husband's arms. At the end of the three days the technician gives me a Certificate for Courage (I kid you not), a CyberKnife key chain (I couldn't make that up), and a big hug (that was great), and tells me to go have a wonderful life.

Can I make it to the meadow myself? (Isaac's question)

Yes, you can and here's how:

- Make a mix tape of one hour of your favorite music.
- Lie down for an hour, don't move, and listen to the music (during a nap, a massage, or while pretending to watch football).

- Picture everyone you've ever loved, hug them, and tell them you love them. Accept their love. While they are there, have fun with them in the ways you most like to have fun.

I'm not sure I signed up for all this meadow stuff. But what happened after CyberKnife? How do you feel now? (Everyone's question.)

Instead of hospital food, we ate at our favorite restaurants. Instead of a hospital bed, we slept in a lovely hotel. Instead of walking the hospital halls with a butt-baring robe and an IV trailing behind, we walked along the bluff in Discovery Park. And instead of visitor's hours, I sat as long as I wanted to in a rocker with Thea and read her stories. Now that it's the day after I am tired and I have a little ache in my shoulder—not worth an aspirin. But I don't have six months of recovery or six months of chemo.

We won't know whether this has worked for 4–6 months so I will sign off from group emails until then, but I love to hear from you so please stay in touch.

Thank you for being at my side.

Love,
Diana

The Waiting Game

Most of us have had an experience of surgery, either personally or vicariously. We expect an operation, an intense period of pain in the hospital, a stretch of bedrest at home, gradual recuperation, and, hopefully, recovery of both mobility and strength. From watching friends or relatives, we also think we know what chemotherapy looks like, even though each drug is different: basically it's hell followed by recovery. But with experimental treatments the aftermath is largely unknown. Dr. Mehta says I may or may not experience fatigue, I may or may not get pneumonitis, and the radiation itself may or may not be effective. The math is pretty simple: I'll know about the fatigue in 2 weeks, the inflammation of lung tissue in

2 months, and the results in 6 months.

Six months? Why so long? We learn that the CT technology that identifies cancer in the first place is fairly worthless for the first six months following intense radiation. Even if the treatment is successful, the radiation will likely leave intensive scarring where the tumor once was, and CTs can't distinguish between scar tissue and cancerous tumor. We hope my body will be effective at disposing of the scar tissue, in which case the mass on the CT will start to shrink over time. Our bigger hope is that the mass won't start to grow again. Any growth would indicate that either the treatment failed, or the gamble of trying a local treatment on a metastatic disease didn't pay off.

So we wait.

⊙ ⊙ ⊙

A little boy's hand reaches up into a tunnel with light at its far end. Camilla's hands reach for his. Behind her are my hands, and the hands of every mother in our ancestral line guiding him to the moment of his birth.

On Saturday, November 17, 2007, Jasper Lindsay Layman was born at his home in Seattle. Camilla had finished up her project at work on Friday; Isaac was almost done with the artwork he was bringing to Miami for a show; and Thea was on her 37th round of singing *Red Red Robin* with Kelly and me. According to the midwives and Jasper's parents, the labor went unusually well; in the time it took Thea, Kel, and me to eat breakfast, fall asleep in the car on a very rainy day, and order a hot dog for lunch, he was born. All nine pounds two ounces of him.

CyberKnife accomplished its goal. Jasper's grandmother is alive, healthy, and strong enough to hold him, softly sing *Tender*

Shepherd, and welcome him into the world. I am thrilled to be able to live my dream of being helpful when little Jasper is born, and the whole family is relieved to turn its attention to holding Jasper, easing Thea's adjustment to a new brother, and helping Camilla recover from the birth. We're all so ready to move back into Normal Life that we move too quickly. Two weeks after Jasper is born, we're on a plane to Miami to see Isaac's art displayed. Two weeks later, Camilla, Thea, and I get pneumonia for Christmas. Camilla ends up being the sickest. We've been so focused on Thea and me that we don't recognize Camilla's blood-oxygen level is dangerously low.

Pneumonia is debilitating and depressing, but in this case it does not become life-threatening, nor does it result in new growth on my scans. At three months they look good, leaving Dr. Mehta cautious but optimistic. Before CyberKnife he had written in my chart that, "there wasn't a lot of evidence that local treatment of metastatic disease would make a difference in the natural history of this disease. The benefit in this particular patient, in these particular conditions is clearly unproven."[40] But he had been willing to try because he believed I'd already made it through what he called "a remarkable stress test," 17 months on Tarceva. Now my response so far to the CyberKnife is another good sign.

Dr. Eaton is cautious but pessimistic, although he would describe it as realistic. In his experience the course of palliative care may be extended, but it only goes one way: downhill. At my checkup he tells me that I don't need a mammogram.

"Why not?"

"Because you have lung cancer."

"But didn't we just treat the cancer? Don't we have to keep a look-out to see if it's elsewhere?"

"You don't need a mammogram."

Oh. Kel and I each do this calculus without speaking. Dr. Eaton still doesn't think I'll live long enough to have to worry about new cancer developing. In his mind, the one I've got is still up to the task of taking me out.

My inner world, however, is not stuck in a six-month waiting game; it is clearly shifting its axis. The celebration in the meadow with our friends' spirits joining me felt more vivid and present than lying still on a table with a linear accelerator whirring above me. It didn't feel like mere imagination; it was somehow a blending of worlds, an exultant and profound experience. And what really blew me away was that Kel had gone there too. When I came out of the second CyberKnife treatment he was in tears in the waiting room. We compared notes over dinner, song by song. What did you see? Who was with you? It was as though we had wandered through the same celebration, fireworks and all. After the party of a lifetime, where do we go from here?

And assuming my dancers had been working to get rid of the cancer, what do they do now if the cancer has indeed been removed? If I see them starting their work up again, does this mean they're just cleaning up after the party, or trying to usher out a new, uninvited guest? Despite all the intimacy we've shared, I admit I'm becoming almost reluctant to see my goddesses. But I still need a way to continue to heal my body, to strengthen the healthy cells' ability to fend off cancer's return, and to clear out the debris and damage from the massive dose of radiation. So I turn to a new way of calming myself during this six-month waiting period.

Extraordinary Knowing: The Power of Qigong

In August I had received a letter from a woman who had gone into remission and wanted to share her success. She had tried one thing that I hadn't yet considered. Qigong is an ancient system of energy medicine that has been practiced in China to prevent disease and treat illness, with documented results. According to an article in the New York Times, "The database of the Qigong Institute includes more than 3,500 studies reporting Qigong's positive effects on hypertension, arthritis, and longevity." But there's a catch. "Rather than randomized controlled studies, the gold standard for Western medicine, many studies are anecdotal, or have small sample sizes."[41] In the absence of hard data, I start looking for a Qigong class.

On Whidbey Island this means recruiting an entire class of students. Once again my friends come through, but at the first class when the instructor, Robert, asked why they were there, they said, "Diana." By the next class (or two, for the diehards) they were all gone.

Qigong to Robert is not a series of yoga poses, nor a martial arts regimen, nor a series of relaxed movements like Tai Chi. Qigong is the study of Qi (or Chi, or Xi, all pronounced "chee"), which is our life force. In class we are going to learn to be like cell phones, tuning in to the frequency that carries the Qi. To sweeten the deal, Robert starts talking about all the extraordinary ways he has seen this information received across time and space. And even though he throws in a detailed scientific descriptions of the mitochondrial energy factories within the cell and how they might be serving as antennae, my western-oriented friends have long since checked out.

But I stay, because it doesn't matter what Robert says, or how he says it. I can feel the Qi, and it feels great. Besides, if I'm aiming for the 1% Club, I'm going to have to keep trying some things that 99% of the population wouldn't. Based on the dropout rate after Robert's first class, Qigong shows promise.

According to Robert, Qigong was passed down as a family secret in China. It was used to train the family's warriors and to heal its members from injury or sickness. Robert teaches a specific form of Qigong called Yi Ren Qigong, developed by Dr. Guan-Cheng Sun based on teachings he learned from his granduncle in China at the age of nine. Trained as a molecular biologist, Dr. Sun combines ancient Chinese wisdom with his western understanding of the cell. I don't understand all the Chinese characters and explanations on his website, but one sentence calls out to me: "The Yi Ren® system of Qigong is designed to support an individual in the exploration and expression of the intelligence and *wisdom already within the body*."

It's very difficult to adequately describe how anything actually feels. My headache, for example, is not anyone else's headache. Even the analogies I might use to describe it—pounding, dull, aching, stabbing—are relevant only to me. So it is with Qi as I experience it in my first class. It feels warm at times, tingling at others. With our eyes closed we move our arms and torsos in very simple movements, not to achieve a desired form or position, like in dance, but to activate energy within the body.[42]

We also work with the idea of an energy field around us, and learn how to clear toxic energy and bring in positive, healing energy. Robert teaches us to consider natural physical phenomena—such as sunlight, water, and wind—as readily available sources of Qi that can be tapped at will to restore different systems within the body. That's the CliffsNotes version, and since it jibes with my own experience, I'm in.

I start Qigong just before the CyberKnife treatment, so between my recovery, Jasper's birth, travelling, and pneumonia my class attendance is sporadic at best. But just because I'm not in class doesn't mean I'm not studying. I've discovered that I can do Qigong meditation anywhere, anytime, without imposing on anyone else. I don't need music, headphones, or even a quiet place to meditate. In fact, I don't need the Qigong movements at all to feel the presence of the Qi, which frees me to practice in bed, on the couch, in line in a grocery store, or sitting on a plane.

Unlike my meditations with the dancers, I don't visualize the actual Qigong movement in my mind. Instead I just feel the result: the energy starts in my abdomen and then moves through my body in the same circuit that it does in class.

It's hard to explain even to myself what this change starts to mean not only in my body but also in the way I view the world. In my long-standing and perfectly serviceable worldview, there was no room for Qigong. Intellectually I can understand that there are, at least at the atomic and molecular level, common building blocks for both living and non-living matter, and that the quest of physics for a unifying principle might one day be realized. I can grasp that there are acknowledged forces that work on everything in the universe. And then into my life comes Qi. It may or may not be part of the electromagnetic spectrum to which we have become accustomed, yet it is now as apparent to me as gravity. But to tell you the truth, at first I wasn't sure if my worldview was cracking open, or if I was cracking up.

This was why I was so primed to read *Extraordinary Knowing: Science, Skepticism and the Inexplicable Powers of the Human Mind* written by a fellow Stanford graduate, Elizabeth Lloyd Mayer. Like me she had had an experience she couldn't rationally explain when a dowser in Alabama was able to locate her daughter's cello in Oakland, California. Instead of shrugging the experience off, Mayer had the courage to seek an explanation. I empathized with her struggles to hold onto both the rational and irrational at once. And I was particularly intrigued by an exchange of emails she had with Garret Yount, a molecular neurobiologist at the California Pacific Medical Center.

Dr. Yount's interest in Qigong began after it helped his father live 13 years with acute leukemia. One of the Qigong masters

Dr. Yount included in his pilot study on distance healing was able to discern from a distance that the culture he had been told contained healthy cells actually contained some healthy cells on top of a bed of culture consisting of thousands of dying cells. This master recognized the presence of unhealthy Qi and worked to eliminate it. None of the other masters did. Yount had controlled for all the variables of the experiment, but he hadn't been able to control for the training each of the masters had received. One's skill level was different. It would be years before I learned that the Qigong master in the experiment was Dr. Sun.

Unfortunately, Qigong is not the only thing I'm struggling to make sense of.

CHAPTER SIX

The Psychology
of Survivorship

January–April, 2008

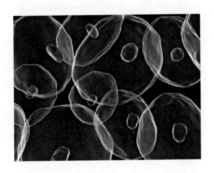

Accoording to the American Cancer Society, 70% of cancer patients fear recurrence.[43] That seems reasonable enough given the high recurrence rates. What doesn't seem reasonable is how overwhelming this fear can become for cancer patients after they've made big strides back to health. Given the certainty of imminent death I had been living with for 21 months, why does this uncertainty bred of hope feel even scarier?

And why do I keep getting so far ahead of myself? It will be another three months before we'll even know if CyberKnife was a game-changer. My mind is torn by cognitive dissonance: either hope predominates or fear rules. Like the Gestalt drawing of either a young woman or a crone depending on how you look at it, I'm having difficulty holding both possibilities in my head simultaneously.

The good three-month scan, while not definitive, has bought me some time—and at the same time it has lowered my psychological defenses. I feel safe enough to be terrified, safe enough to finally cry. And I want to do it with Sarri Gilman, the therapist who has helped me when I've needed it most.

"Cancer can open up some very dark places, Diana," Sarri affirms when we meet. "This is normal, and it may not be possible to get rid of this anxiety altogether. But we can take the poison out of it. You're holding a trunk full of unexpressed fear, tears, and emotions. So let's unpack them—safely."

At the beginning of every doctor visit, regardless of hospital or clinic, a nurse weighs me, takes my blood pressure and temperature, and asks me to rate my pain on a scale of 1 to 10. If I have trouble navigating the ten-point scale, there are unhappy and happy faces in both English and Spanish available to guide me. Anxiety has a scale just like pain does. Mercifully, I usually answer the nurse with a zero when she asks about my pain. Anxiety, however, has been my daily companion, sitting lightly on my shoulder waiting to spring into action or rooted so deep in my solar plexus that it's difficult to breathe.

In our previous session Sarri suggested that the ways I had dealt with anxiety before were largely to push it away or stomp it out. This time she has asked me to listen to anxiety's messages by personifying her, by capitalizing her name just as I first personified Lung Woman in my first meditation. What does Anxiety look like? I laugh at my first image. She's a two-year-old like Thea—who in these first months after Jasper's birth can go from zero to sixty in one second. But today, as I pay attention to the way Anxiety spends her time with me, she starts to seem older, more nuanced, a young woman perhaps. What role is she playing? After watching the various ways she interacts with me, and listening to her messages, I make a list.

Anxiety is:

- *An alarm clock and reminder button.* Did you take your Tarceva today?
- *A watchdog/vigilante/personal trainer.* Be careful, are you watching what you're eating? Did you exercise today? Are you staying with the program?
- *A brake.* Careful, don't take on too much.
- *A dispatcher for the immune system,* sending out the search parties to see whether invaders lurk anywhere in its territory.

This last one fascinates me. In the same way that discontent drives me to learn, could anxiety lead me to heal? Perhaps those search parties include T-cells, the immune system's police force, that mature in the thymus, the organ in the chest between the breastbone and heart—exactly the area that gets tight when I'm anxious. What I most fear is that Anxiety is prescient, that every time she bellows she does so because she *knows* something is wrong. But if her role is to organize shift schedules rather than read the future, Anxiety isn't necessarily responding to a specific 911 call from a crime in progress. Instead, she might be sending T-cells on routine patrols to a neighborhood that my immune system has targeted as high-crime. Since the cancer was originally able to get a foothold because my immune system didn't recognize cancerous cells as invaders, isn't this a big step forward?

When I tell Kelly about all this, he has the massage table and a candle burning and gives me a treatment that takes all the remaining stress away. I invite Anxiety to join the healing circle as a Goddess-in-Training. When I tell Sarri, she suggests I make a deal with my inner healers: Let the predictive role of Crystal Ball Gazer reside in the exclusive domain of the medical community. Now that I'm getting plenty of CTs and MRIs to keep us abreast of what's what, the goddesses don't have to carry that load anymore.

The Futility of Moat-Building

Qigong as a calming agent is not working. Politely allowing Anxiety to join the party is not working. I'm crying. My question is not *where do I find bliss today?* but *how do I hold onto life?* Waiting has turned into wandering in the wilderness. I'm not in the healing glen, and I feel lost.

 I am trying to climb up out of a steep Utah slot canyon. I feel vulnerable on the canyon walls, not only because I'm not trained in climbing and I'm not sure I have the strength, but also because I feel like the talus slopes of cancer could cause me to slip and fall at any moment.

I've got heavy ropes around my waist that I'm not using properly. Instead of attaching them to a pulley or a climbing harness, I'm dragging them up from the canyon floor. Their weight exhausts me as I climb, and their length makes it seem like it's only a matter of time before they get caught on something and pull me down to the valley floor.

I'm not using the ropes. They're using me.

Climbing up loose rock is not the image I'm craving right now. I want Stress Chick thrown out by the nearest bouncer. I want Bubble Girl to invite me into her bullet-proof, germ-proof, Teflon-coated, stress-free, impermeable home. But what good is living in a fortress if the invader is already inside the walls?

Yesterday Sarri suggested that I try to understand what I'm so anxious about. What am I trying to protect myself from? Duh. This is so obvious, why are we even having this discussion? I fidget and rearrange the pillows on the leather couch. "I'm afraid of dying a very painful death. What's there to learn from that?" There, I said it, but that's as close to talking about death as I can go, and mercifully the session is almost over. So Sarri gives me homework.

Today I sit down with a blank piece of paper in front of me, label it *Protection*, and start drawing in the hope that my right brain will find an answer that eludes my left. I draw Death in the upper right corner along with its minion, Pain, and draw a pitiful two-brick-high wall in the lower left corner to protect me from them. But I gain new understanding as I draw three paths in the middle of the page that I am afraid will lead me directly there—*Sorrow, Illness,* and *Stress.*

Sorrow is the flash flood that feels like it will sweep me off the canyon walls and carry me crashing against the rocks downstream. The floodwaters are tears of my fellow survivors—their feelings of hopelessness, depression, anger, and grief—along with the overwhelming sadness that I'm starting to feel from a crisis brewing in our extended family. I feel like I'm taking sorrow in but I can't expel it; this won't help anyone, especially me.

I'm also afraid of *Illness*, the storm developing around me, an outside element like cold, flu, or pneumonia that could weaken my immune system. Thea and Jasper are the proverbial canaries in the mine—the first to get any virus that passes through Seattle; when is the exact moment I'm supposed to leave them, or stay home, to minimize my exposure?

The third path is *Stress*. Not all stress is unhealthy. Healthy stress strengthens our bones by depositing layers of calcium, and lack of healthy stress weakens them.[44] Too much stress, however, and they break. I grew up skiing as close to straight down the mountain as I could come. It was exhilarating to face mogul after mogul while singing a song to keep me in rhythm. As Kelly and I grew our business, I didn't pay much attention when my friends would counsel me about stress. Every new product we offered represented something I had never done before. I liked the sensation of challenging myself and discovering I was capable. And I knew people in much more stressful jobs than mine who were doing fine.

I've always thought stress was something I could handle. But judging by the cancer, perhaps my body thinks differently. By 2008 the impact of stress on the body is well researched and widely publicized. Stress chemicals are designed to increase alertness so you can recognize a threat, increase blood flow to the muscles so you make a swift get-away, and even dull your pain receptors so you can continue to run if you're injured. The problem is, in stressful times those parts of the body that the brain believes aren't critical get reduced resources. Growth, reproduction, and, most importantly for me now, the immune system, are put on hold.

And unfortunately the source of the threat doesn't have to be a saber-tooth tiger—our minds are quite capable of inventing danger, thank you very much.

Scientists have found the link between psychological stress and immuno-suppression in the form of a neuropeptide that interferes with immune defenses.[45] This has convinced me that stress *is* toxic to me. I have already cleared out the obvious stresses from work and community service, but the imagery in my climbing meditation suggests that it's not an outer source of stress that I'm worried about today. It's the damn ropes. And they're mine. They are my own patterns of thinking, my own learned behaviors that I'm still dragging around, and they are exhausting. I've got to either take them off or transform them into something useful.

Psychologist Susan Vaughn has said "an effective psychotherapist is a 'microsurgeon of the mind' who helps patients make needed alterations in neuronal networks."[46] Today Sarri and I are making those alterations from a vantage point deep within my psyche. Sarri would later compare this session to a high-wire act, the two of us crossing a cable stretched hundreds of feet off the ground, traversing the canyon from one way of viewing my life to another.

I start the session by talking about how depleted I feel when Kel and I visit my mother's house. In other words, I start with the mother lode of patterns. These days I no longer have the energy to play mediator in family conflicts, a role I assigned myself early in life. I no longer feel that it's safe for me to be in the middle of anyone else's fight with my mother—their anger and frustration exhausts me, and I feel too much of the pain my mother doesn't express. And because I have already tied in with a mental rope of causality—*stress leads to illness, leads to cancer returning, leads to pain, leads to death*—the more stress I feel, the more I fear my cancer returning.

"Does anyone want you to feel exhaustion, Diana?" Sarri gently asks.

"No."

"Does anyone want you to sacrifice your health for them?"

This is it. The most toxic pattern. As a culture, we revere the person who runs into a wall of flames to save a child, who jumps into the river to save a drowning person. Mothers, of course, do it all the time when their children are very young, sacrificing their own sleep and health to care for their infant. Wasn't this behavior worth emulating? But for me, this pattern of responsibility for others has gone beyond being an older sister, a mother, a community volunteer, and even the president of a company. Long ago I allowed my body to be used to save another's, and then I did my best to carry on with my life as if this had never happened. It was the buried root of this pattern that made it so poisonous.

Sarri and I start to examine my every relationship for signs of the ropes, for old ways of being. We aren't looking for in-depth psychotherapy, we want to extract the nectar and move on. Do I want my mother to listen to me as a child in need of attention, or as a grown daughter concerned about her health? Am I reacting as an older sister who wants to protect a sibling from frustration, or as a peer who is there to listen? Do I want to rescue my colleagues at work by taking on a project even when I know it's taking precious time away from my healing?

As we quickly move through each relationship I can see that the stress I feel comes from wanting life to be different than it is, from wanting someone else to be other than they are, of wanting those relationships to be what they aren't. But then I realize that the hardest work is to recognize that I want to be someone I'm not. I want to have not done the things I wish I hadn't, and to have done what I wished I had: as a daughter, a sibling, a friend, a wife, a mother, and an executive. I want to be someone who doesn't have shame, guilt, and confusion. I want to be someone who has answers for other survivors that I don't have for myself.

"Diana, you've spent nearly two years listening closely to your body," continues Sarri. "How does it feel when you don't listen to it and it gets depleted?"

"Betrayed."

"Is it reasonable to ask of yourself what you can't reasonably do?" she asks.

"You mean, what good is being angry and disappointed with myself over a past that can't be changed, a present I can't understand, and a future that might not happen?"

I start laughing. And then I'm laughing so hard I can't speak, releasing some of the stress of demanding the undoable. I recognize that I have to treat myself with the same love I give to others and they give me. My body's advice is: Let go of the heavy ropes. Forgive yourself.

$$\odot \odot \odot$$

When did I first hear the phrase, "Use it or lose it?" My memory serves up light-blue polyester track-suits, so I'm guessing a gym in the late 1970s. I associate the maxim with things I don't want to lose: lift weights so you don't lose muscle; do crossword puzzles so you don't lose brain cells. But brain research reveals that the corollary is also true. "Unlearning and weakening connections between neurons is … just as important as learning and strengthening them," reported Dr. Norman Doidge in his mind-bending book, *The Brain That Changes Itself: Stories of Personal Triumph From the Frontiers of Brain Science.*[47] In fact, to make way for the new we often have to lose the old, which is why it's easier to learn French in France when you're not speaking English all the time. Learning a new pattern of thinking requires a disruption in our normal patterns. Certainly cancer propelled me to let go of outer stress. Now the hope of surviving it is the catalyst for taking on my inner stress.

So as soon as I recognize what's happening I stop myself from firing patterns that produce stress, guilt, inner conflict, outer obligation, or just plain meddling. At first this is a lot of work. If I find myself in someone else's shoes, trying to take their stress—or learning opportunity—away from them, or giving them something I think they need without letting them first ask for my help, I retreat to my own boundaries. I have no control over their world anyway, and increasingly I recognize that I have no right to be there either. I not only stop giving my opinion, I practice not having the opinion in the first place. Within myself, I re-affirm that I will listen first of all to my body's requirements and honor my need to get the exercise, sleep, and nutrition I require, before committing to anything else—even to being with the grandchildren I adore.

Embracing the Unknown

Repatterning is a lot easier than I expected. I love my family and friends, and they are not the problem: I am, and I'm motivated to change. Practice may not make perfect, but it's close enough. It's harder to let go of my mental constructs of *stress leads to illness, leads to cancer returning, leads to pain, leads to death* and the shorter string: *stage 4 lung cancer leads to imminent death.* Fortunately this logic is tied together by easily unraveled granny knots, as Sarri quickly points out.

"How do you know that this path is inevitable, or that the cause-and-effect links are even true?" She points out that my doctors might be bright, well-intentioned, and empathetic, but they are not prophets. Certainly all of them had been wrong about the timing of my death. She helps me untangle everything that doctors, alternative healers, well-meaning friends, books, magazines, or websites have said to me, and we place each bit of counsel into one of two piles: "The Known," and "The Unknown." The Known pile ends up being remarkably small. Not only is there not much evidence that applies to me, there don't seem to be many other survivors to emulate. Sarri reminds me, "There is the '*known* unknown' and there is the '*unknown* unknown.' I don't think you can trust that any claim made with absolute certainty will be right for you." This helps me close the window on a lot of websites.

For homework I consider why the concept of known and unknown resonates so keenly with me. Why have I let Dr. Eaton's view of the Known World of Stage 4 Lung Cancer (that Death's save-the-date card may have been premature, but a new one will be in the mail soon) invade my every thought? What is about white lab coats that is so spell-binding? Before this cancer, I had no reason to question Western medicine. In fact I was one of its cheerleaders, grateful for its cure of my colon cancer, and confident that its inexorable push for knowledge would help me with whatever might ail me whenever I needed it.

But now all the knowledge accumulated by decades of perseverance and dedication on the part of countless doctors, surgeons, and researchers, is still coming up short for me. What oncologists know is that their stage 4 lung cancer patients die. This happens all the time at major cancer centers, and I'm sure that only by not getting his expectations too high can Dr. Eaton come into work every day without being overcome by depression. I can understand how this might be a great strategy for him, but it's not a great one for me.

I am ready to hike into the unknown. As massive, unsettling, mind-bending, and illusion-shattering as it might be, it is still a friendlier place for me to roam than the alternative. Sarri has just given me a new map, and as I turn it to orient myself, I feel my whole spirit pivoting from a world where only 1% survive to a world where 1% is what we know and 99% is what we still have to learn. It seems like everywhere I look, in just about any field, I see members of this 1% is What We Know Club.

Take physics: "We can now say what the main ingredients of the universe are: it's made of 4% atoms, about 25% dark matter, and 71% mysterious dark energy latent in empty space. That's settled a question that we've wondered about, certainly the entire 35 years I've been doing cosmology,"[48] says Sir Martin Rees, Royal Society Professor at Cambridge University. That's settled? But we don't even know what dark matter is, much less the mysterious dark energy. And there are still holes in what we know about the 4% that's left!

Or listen to Stanford's Dean of Engineering: "We're only just beginning to turn biology into a science that can be applied in the way that chemistry, mathematics and physics have been applied."[49] Just beginning? Then why is Kel's biology degree from that same institution 35 years ago a Bachelor's of *Science*?

On the other hand, I am taken with what Harvard psychology professor Daniel Gilbert says in his book *Stumbling on Happiness*: "Our ability to simulate future selves and future circumstances is by no means perfect. When we imagine future circumstances, we fill in details that won't really come to pass and leave out details that will. When we imagine future feelings, we find it impossible to ignore what we are feeling now and impossible to recognize how we will think about the things that happen later."[50] And I am smitten with Gregory Cochran, adjunct professor of anthropology at the University of Utah, who says, "There is something new under the sun—us."[51] As a species, our brains continue to change and evolve.

I'm seeing that it's not just a question of how little we know, it's also that so much of what we think we know is wrong. Surprisingly, this new perspective isn't turning me away from science; it's drawing me toward it. Living with the unknown can be transformative. Like the bumper sticker implies, not believing everything I think can be liberating. And just because something is unknown—or unproven—as a strategy for fighting stage 4 lung cancer doesn't mean it hasn't been established and explored at length within its own field, as is the case with dream analysis, for example.

My job is to make new connections, or to find a way to experiment with existing ones. There are areas like neuroscience where new trails are being blazed daily, and in these cases I'm trying to build a bridge from the theoretical to something I can use right now. And I don't forget that someday one of those scientists working late into the night could turn a hunch into a reality, and save my life.

It boils down to this: as long as the first question I ask myself each morning is "How do I protect myself from death?" the answer is going to be stressful. So I stop thinking about survival as a scramble up a steep, slippery slope back to the life I'd known, and start to think about its root, *sur-vivere*—living beyond—and of joyfully, exuberantly, striding straight out of the canyon into the unknown, with Kelly, my healing team, my family, and my friends by my side.

I don't know if it's the Ghost of Shaman Past or Survivor Guilt that is hijacking my dreams, but I'm obsessing over my life's purpose. What is the purpose of any life, after all is said and done? Is it to love as whole-heartedly as I can? To learn as courageously and open-mindedly as possible? Or is it to give back—even if only a fraction of what I've received?

"Let's drink to little goals," our friends Debora and Steve suggest over dinner. It's a start.

The next week, Shoshana, my patient coordinator in Dr. Eaton's office, is checking the system to make my next appointment. She looks up from her computer.

"Why do you think you're doing so well?" she asks.

"Love," I answer.

She takes her hands off her keyboard. Her head slightly tilted, she asks, "Do you *really* start each day by thinking about where you're going to find some love?"

"I do."

She is silent but she looks straight into me. I can almost hear the vow she is making to herself.

⊙ ⊙ ⊙

A side trail off a beach in Santa Barbara leads me to a little cove, its sand revealed by the outgoing tide, its rocks sheltering me with privacy. I drink in its sublime beauty, close my eyes to heighten the sound of waves, and bask in the warmth of the sun. I'm aware that my senses aren't just delivering information, they're triggering a flood of chemicals throughout my body. I feel my pores open to receive sunshine, bits of immortal information flowing to my cells. I can feel the power of the moon on my inner oceans, tugging the toxins out with the tide.

One stringed instrument in a very large orchestra, I am gloriously and vibrantly alive—a fact made all the more poignant because I am here today to celebrate the life of my friend Carolyn who has just died of cancer. It's the first time I've been away from Kel since my own diagnosis, yet I feel such a strong connection to him that the miles have no meaning. I never expected when I got married that I would be this much in love 33 years later. My love for my children, children-in-law, and grandchildren also reside deep in my body. Aren't these feelings of joy far more than I could reasonably ask of a lifetime, however long?

On the way home, during a layover in the Portland airport, I happen upon a *Wall Street Journal* article about the latest research into love. Researchers already know that romantic love generates endorphins and dopamine, chemicals that overwhelm the reasoning parts of the brain and stimulate the regions that govern addiction. Today the big news is that a group of researchers has found couples who have sustained this state of romantic love for decades.[52] I'm one of them! I'm standing in the middle of the concourse, travelers streaming by, wanting to yell out like Gene Kelly on the lamppost in *Singin' in the Rain* that I'm *in* love with Kelly again. More common at our age are the love-in-the-long-run chemicals, oxytocin and vasopressin, which are better suited to building and sustaining a lifelong relationship. Kelly and I have these, too, but we're definitely taking a refresher course in Romance Chemistry 101. Both sets of chemicals are great. But one is chocolate-and-roses; the other is chocolate-and-roses-can-wait.

According to Dr. Louann Brizendine's book, *The Female Brain*, "Mother love looks a lot like romantic love on a brain scan … switching on pleasure circuits that produce feelings of exhilaration and attachment."[53] What about grandmother love? When I think of all my friends who are new grandparents, I know we must be generating goofy chemicals too. Why else would we incessantly look at pictures of our grandchildren, chuckle when we tell stories about them, and rush to their side whenever we can? Friendship must generate variations in this chemistry too. It's hard to believe this chemistry of love isn't having a tonic effect on my immune system, and in fact I find studies linking dopamine and oxytocin to increased immune response.[54]

Love has another benefit. Neuroscientists are discovering that our brains are never too old to change, a quality they called plasticity. What chemical promotes this ability to make new neuronal connections? Oxytocin—the hormone of love! Researchers have found that oxytocin plays a key role in nature when mothers need to be able to change their brain patterns in order to un-bond from the first litter in order to bond with the next.[55] Maybe the Beatles were right: All you *do* need is love.

What can I use this new brain for? Well, I've spent the 18 months after diagnosis following my bliss, and now I want to understand how the components of bliss that so enriched my emotional and spiritual wellness might also have contributed to my body's health. If love has changed the chemistry of my body and the pathways of my brain, what about everything else I've tried? Serendipitously, every day brings me new ideas to research. Today, for example, a friend has sent an email about a study featured in the May 2007 *Scientific American*[56] that finds the optimal moment of plasticity is right after some new connection is made. New neurons are constantly being formed in an adult brain and they have a two-week window during which they are optimally primed to learn.[57]

"It seems that for high levels of plasticity what matters is the age of the single neuron and not the age of the brain," says Tommaso Pizzorusso, a neurobiologist at the Institute of Neuroscience of the National Research Council in Pisa, Italy.[58] So I'm quickly acting on new healing ideas before the opportunity to leverage the power of that neuron dies. In our globally-connected culture, an email leads to a web search leads to a conversation, synapse to synapse to synapse. But what has changed for me over these last two years is that I no longer want to merely understand a concept, I want to try it out in my body. I am expanding my initial strategy of *listen and respond;* now it's becoming *seek, try, listen, and respond.* And as I take on this new intention, my pace of discovery accelerates.

Sarri says watching me is like playing old 33 ⅓ LPs on 78.

I start this day wondering whether music, like love, also releases chemicals that could fortify my immune system. So I call a friend who's a music therapist and invite her for lunch to discuss the connection between music and healing. After lunch, she teaches me how to tone—how to improvise together using only vowel sounds. Researchers have found that when humans tone, sing, or chant together, our bodies respond and synchronize: our heart rhythms move from "chaos," the rhythm of stress, anxiety, depression and anger, to "coherence," the state of well-being, compassion, and gratitude—and our hearts literally beat as one.[59]

I love the idea of coherence and I wonder where it will lead me. I experiment during a massage to see if silently toning can be as effective as toning out loud, and whether parts of my body beside my heart can move into the same state of coherence.

"Where did you go today in your meditation? I was able to go much deeper into your fascia layers," says Jill, after the massage is over. A new idea has manifested in my body. And I want to explore another one tomorrow: "Introducing young neurons," says senior study author Hongjun Song, an assistant professor of neurology at Johns Hopkins University School of Medicine in Baltimore, "can make the older circuitry more plastic and adapt to new conditions."[60] I figure this is the role that Thea and Jasper, their bodies bursting with new neurons, play in my older circuitry. So I spend the next day with my two-year old granddaughter. Our destination is the lake, but we never make it. Instead, we spend an hour in the grassy strip between the sidewalk and the street outside Thea's house. The songs we make up together, using leaves, branches, and seeds as our percussion section, delight us no end.

If you want to know what it's like to spend a day living in the now, spend it with a two-year old. Not the way we do when

we're parenting, but when we're grandparenting: fully letting
go of our own agenda in order to embrace the toddler's world.
In young children, the learning switch is continuously turned on.[61]
They focus on everything because they don't yet have a bias about
what is worth paying attention to. In my drive to understand what
has contributed to my healing, I'm trying to let go of my biases
too. And I'm discovering that the process of searching, trying,
listening to my body, and adapting my response accordingly,
makes my days not only joyful but downright fascinating.

Over dinner one night, a friend wonders whether she has
to wait to get sick in order to enjoy some of this. Another friend
points out that any of us could have chosen to spend this Saturday
ambling on a beach singing to themselves, as I did. But Kel offers
another possibility, making an analogy to chaparral, the tough
scrubby plants that literally have to go through fire to crack open
their seeds. "I think we might need the fire, too," he says. "Maybe
it takes something that intense to break open our shells and start
us growing again."

Speaking the Language of Cells

Island living teaches us that regardless of where we want to go, we
are not always in control of when we get to start our trip. Our ferry
lines are a metaphor for the illusion of a planned life. We each have
personal strategies for how we'll use these random gifts of time
provided by one, two, and three-boat waits. If the line starts on the
final descent to the tollbooth, there's time enough to recline our
seats and savor the gorgeous panorama of the waters, mountains,
and islands of Puget Sound. But for times when the line snakes
far up the hill where the tall Douglas firs obscure the view, many
of us keep a book tucked away.

Mine today is by Deepak Chopra, which I've picked up at a used bookstore. "The body is not a frozen sculpture," he writes. "It is a river of information—a flowing organism empowered by millions of years of intelligence … You believe that you live in the world when in fact the world lives in you."[62]

Only a few pages in, I close my eyes and am sucked into a meditation.

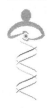

A powerful, cascading current carries me downriver, over waterfalls and into deep warm pools of energy in my body, from lungs to heart to solar plexus. Two parallel rivers rush, flush, and cleanse all the water molecules in their incessant and rhythmic circuit up my spine and down the front of my torso.

I pick up a telescope that combines the characteristics of both the Hubble Space Telescope and electron microscopy. The scope focuses on one of my cells, a glass sphere as vast as the universe. It is stunningly beautiful in both its complexity and simplicity. I am deeply grateful to the cell for revealing itself to me.

I can see through and beyond the cell into the cosmos of my body, populated by countless cells going about their business, oblivious to my observation. One of the cells slightly shifts in the corner of my eye, then crosses my field of vision like a shooting star pulled to an unknown destination. I witness another cell splitting in two. Many cells remain relatively stable, allowing me an unhurried and unimpeded opportunity to observe them.

I'm still distantly aware of conversations around me in the ferry lot. I feel the car rock as Kel gets out and returns with hot chocolate, I hear the ignitions of the cars around us starting, and keep my balance as the car rumbles over the ramp into the boat, but I don't want to come out of this trance. The irresistible imagery holds me captive, and draws me into a deeper hypnotic state. I even hold my breath so as to not jostle my mind. The images are so breathtaking, the intelligence within the body so vivid, that I find myself thinking it's almost worth getting cancer just to experience this, if only once in a lifetime.

This meditation triggers my awe, wonder, and gratitude for the infinite vastness of a cell. Like a beginners foreign language class my meditation uses minimal vocabulary, in this case to describe three basic states of a cell: a seemingly stable cell that reveals its inner workings to me, a shifting state where the cell is in motion, and a cell in the act of replicating. I'm as excited as an astronomer who after decades of peering through a telescope finally witnesses a star being born, and as the images slip from my grasp, I hold my focus long enough to hear, "We're always here. You can come back whenever you want."

"You've learned to talk cell," says Sarri. I've brought up my ferry line experience in the hope that she can ground me, but instead she's suggesting I'm in completely new territory. This data does not fit my hypothesis of how the world works, and yet her explanation seems to describe exactly what's happening—not at my conscious instigation, but bubbling up from some deeper level of being. I've come this far talking to myself, so why stop now? If I don't open myself up to this new knowledge, then I might miss a huge opportunity.

Researchers know that cells communicate laterally, that is, with each other; I had suspected that perhaps what I was seeing in my inner images was my body trying to communicate directly with me, but I'm still stunned by how specific the messages are getting! And my vision/meditations seem to be increasingly refined. We've moved from goddesses to organs to cells being acted upon to the inner world of the cells themselves.

⊙ ⊙ ⊙

Jill Bolte Taylor's TED talk reaches me through an email forward. A neuroanatomist by training, Taylor was able to recognize the events of the morning she had a stroke in her left brain *while it was happening.* What captivates me is the story of the peace, connectedness, and bliss she felt in her right brain once her left brain was silenced.

> I can no longer define the boundaries of my body. I can't define where I begin and where I end. Because the atoms and the molecules of my arm blended with the atoms and molecules of the wall. And all I could detect was this energy. Energy.[63]

I am not alone in these experiences I'm having. My experience during my visualizations is a lighter shade of pale next to hers, but it's there nonetheless. Taylor's experience encourages me to believe I've reached the right side of my brain after all—blessedly without having a stroke. Her insight must have inspired my cells as well, because I quickly get another glimpse of them.

As I lie down and enter my inner world, I see the three types of cells from the earlier meditation: the stable, the shifting, and the replicating. Like a tigress pouncing on a kill, the main healer rushes into the dividing cells and holds them vice-like while she wraps them in what at first seems like a hard plastic wrap. But something about the hardness of this material does not seem right to her. The image zooms as the healer transforms the wrap into a softer, yet impenetrable goo. Goo? I think to myself. Yes, definitely goo.

While this image is crystal clear, my ability to translate this into a biological principle is not. Goo? How can I possibly find out what this means? It turns out I only have to go as far as an article in *Cure* magazine that's sitting in Dr. Eaton's waiting room. The title of the article, "Medicine's New Epicenter? Epigenetics" wouldn't have caught my eye but the cover illustration—a light switch in the middle of DNA strands—reminded me of a meditation of hands rapidly switching black cells to white cells. The subtitle of the article—"New field of epigenetics may hold the secret to flipping cancer's 'off' switch"—provides a possible explanation of my inner imagery and entices me to keep reading.

We know that we all inherit a genetic code. The goal of gene therapy research has been to identify the specific genetic mutation for a given disease and then target therapies only to those genes, leaving the healthy parts of the cell untouched. However, so far targeted therapies haven't delivered much on the promise of personalized medicine made at the start of the Human Genome Project.[64] A single link between one gene and one disease, like that between the inherited BCRA-1 gene and breast cancer, is the rare exception.

Unfortunately, cancer cells are usually much more creative in the ways they create and commandeer resources. The drug I'm taking, Tarceva, blocks the signaling pathway of a single mutation in the EGFR/HER1 receptor. Tarceva typically fails because the cancer eventually finds a work-around to get what it needs. (To make the situation even more daunting, in 2010, Zemin Zhang, a senior scientist from Genentech, the company that makes Tarceva, will discover 50,000 mutations in the tumor of a heavy smoking lung cancer patient.[65] How do you deal with that?)

Scientists at the time were finding that genes were not the whole story because "the genetic coding of a malignant cell often appeared to be, by all appearances, normal."[66] There was something impacting how the genes work and are passed down that didn't involve changing their DNA sequence. The study of these factors is called epigenetics, named for traits that exist "on top of" or "in addition to" genetics.[67] The *Cure* article described our genes as the blueprint for how our cells manufacture proteins, and our epigenes as the contractor that decides how that blueprint is actually used, and gets the necessary materials to do the building.

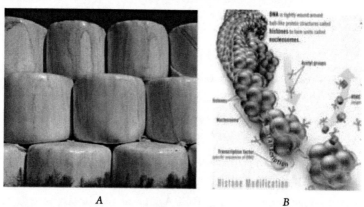

A   B

Figure 2. Epigenetics. In my meditation, the cell was wrapped too tightly like a hay bale wrapped in plastic (A). In some cancers, the DNA *is* wrapped too tightly around a histone, preventing the tumor suppressor gene from doing its job (B). Epigenetic researchers are trying to develop a new class of drugs to correct this.

One way the epigenetic layer can go awry is if the DNA is wound too tightly around a ball-like protein structure called a histone, effectively turning off the tumor suppressor gene. This is the part of the article that reminds me of the hard plastic that needed to soften into "goo" in my meditation. Perhaps I need to "loosen" the wrapping so my tumor suppressor genes can turn on and read their instructions properly.

I file the word "epigenetics" away in my brain. If epigenetic therapy is ever presented to me as an option, it might be worth considering.

Giving back: Can I Share What I'm Doing Right?

Eighteen months after my original diagnosis I'm also asking myself, what *is* that something I'm doing *right*? It's starting to haunt me. I've moved from relief at my own reprieve to a sense of obligation to help others. Have I inadvertently stumbled across something that could be replicated, or is my health simply the result of a freakishly lucky genetic fit with Tarceva? If there is something that someone else could use, what is it? I feel a tremendous urgency because some of my fellow cancer survivors are dying.

I start where Dr. Eaton began: single-agent Tarceva is not enough on its own to cure me. So regardless of whether we think it has carried 50%, 75%, or even 99% of the workload in my particular case, there is still x% unaccounted for. It's possible that CyberKnife took care of that remaining percentage and that Western medicine has been the total answer. But Tarceva's track record isn't that good, and CyberKnife in the thoracic cavity doesn't have much of a record at all.

So what accounts for the remaining x-factor? Maybe everything we've been doing *is* helping Tarceva reach its target. I can see from the simulation video on the Genentech site that many of the golden Tarceva molecules flying toward the cell bounced off without landing where they were supposed to (see figure 3). Have my love chemicals created a highway, a beacon, or a starship that help Tarceva reach the EGFR/HER1 receptor in the tumor cells with greater frequency and accuracy?

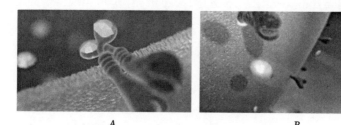

A   *B*

Figure 3. Tarceva landing on the HER-1 receptor. Has everything I've done helped me to better deliver and absorb the Tarceva to the EGFR/HER1 receptor (A) instead of having the Tarceva bounce off the cell (B)?

But I can also see from the video that there are many ways that the tumor grows, so perhaps there are many ways of disrupting this process. Was it possible that everything I experienced created additional chemicals or forces, matter or energy, which acted independently or together against the cancer cells? Or somehow changed the neighborhood the tumor cells lived in so that it was less attractive, maybe even hostile? If so, how effective was each individual agent in boosting the immune system and/or fighting the cancer?

Faced with all these questions I do what every marketer does in the absence of hard data or available product: I create a PowerPoint presentation (see figure 4). I attempt to extract reason from mystery. I list the chemicals I've discovered that are released by love and music, knowing that some of them have already been shown to boost the immune system.[68] I add in new research on the benefits of exercise in combination with cancer treatment; we know that chemicals released in exercise also boost the immune system, but how much exercise is needed to battle a stage 4 tumor load? If all these chemicals are relevant, how powerful is the booster shot?

What about the power of synergy? Does 1+1=3 when multiple agents work in combination? There are thousands of receptors on each tumor cell. If we imagine Tarceva plugging up receptors 1–10, was music responsible for ports 11–13, and exercise for 14–18? What about the even less quantifiable elements, like prayer, placebo, and pink bracelets? Exactly how much are twenty hugs, four miles of walking, a fruit smoothie, and twenty minutes of laughter worth in overcoming any given day's disease burden? While my mind is obsessing over this puzzle, my body feels like a human petri dish, an important lab experiment in which I can change my own parameters and do my own trial.

The idea that beauty, friendship, gratitude, love, and laughter are not just part of appreciating each day but are in fact medicine as important as Tarceva, supplements, or Asian mushrooms, enriches my minutes, hours, days, and months and leads to a deep sense of well-being. If I could feel this way each day, then perhaps the number of days I had left was ultimately beside the point.

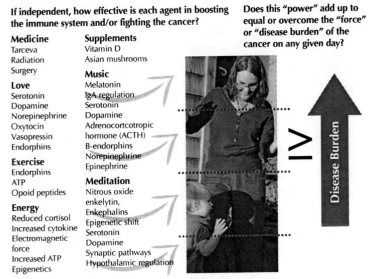

If independent, how effective is each agent in boosting the immune system and/or fighting the cancer?

Does this "power" add up to equal or overcome the "force" or "disease burden" of the cancer on any given day?

Medicine
Tarceva
Radiation
Surgery

Love
Serotonin
Dopamine
Norepinephrine
Oxytocin
Vasopressin
Endorphins

Exercise
Endorphins
ATP
Opoid peptides

Energy
Reduced cortisol
Increased cytokine
Electromagnetic force
Increased ATP
Epigenetics

Supplements
Vitamin D
Asian mushrooms

Music
Melatonin
IgA regulation
Serotonin
Dopamine
Adrenocortcotropic hormone (ACTH)
B-endorphins
Norepinephrine
Epinephrine

Meditation
Nitrous oxide
enkelytin,
Enkephalins
Epigenetic shift
Serotonin
Dopamine
Synaptic pathways
Hypothalamic regulation

Disease Burden

Figure 4. Can anything I'm doing help others?

As excited as I am by the thought that what I'm learning

could at least initiate a conversation that might be helpful to someone else, I am overwhelmed by the responsibility: what if what I suggest proves harmful? How could what I'm discovering be supported by research? Studies are designed to evaluate one or two parameters. How was anyone going to make up a clinical trial group of 56 grandmothers in their mid-fifties who were being treated for lung cancer? Double that number to test for Vitamin D. Double again for exercise. And again for love of music. It was an unlikely scenario, to say the least. And it called into doubt, for me, any clinical trial that tested for a single factor. Of the terminal patients in a given study, how many even had a strong will to live?

Actually I later learned that even the single variable studies are often flawed. Author and journalist David Freedman started to "…examine why expert pronouncements so often turn out to be exaggerated, misleading, or flat-out wrong."[69] He found a 2005 study by John Ioannidis of the University of Ioannina in Greece that "examined the 45 most prominent studies published since 1990 in the top medical journals and found that about one-third of them were ultimately refuted. If one were to look at all medical studies, it would be more like two-thirds, [Ioannidis] says. And for some kinds of leading-edge studies, like those linking a disease to a specific gene, wrongness infects 90 percent or more." One example was the Women's Health Initiative that discovered that the routinely prescribed hormone replacement therapy not only didn't benefit against heart disease, it increased the risk of stroke and cancer.[70]

I wonder whether the term evidence-based medicine is overstating the case. Freedman postulates that this problem occurs largely because of what he calls "the streetlight effect."

"Large, clean studies can take years of planning, fund raising, and lining up patients, plus a decade or more to execute. That is why we first get bombarded by years of weaker studies plagued by the streetlight effect—looking for answers where the looking is good, rather than where the answers are likely to be hiding."[71]

And what about the 860 cancer drugs currently in trial—of which only two will ultimately make it to market this year?[72] I, like most cancer patients, don't have years to wait for researchers to quit duking it out and arrive at a verdict, not to mention the 17 years it typically takes to get a drug from "laboratory bench to bedside."[73] We're in the process of betting our lives on every pill we take or don't take, every procedure we attempt or don't try, and every action or inaction we put our body through. And we usually have little evidence as a basis for our decisions.

Sarri laughs when I show her my PowerPoint and excitedly point to the diagram of everything I think has helped me get to where I am today (see figure 5).

My healing plan (April 2006–April 2008)

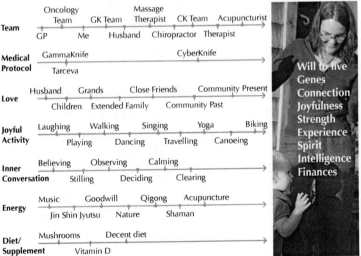

Team	Oncology Team, GK Team, Massage Therapist, CK Team, Acupuncturist		
	GP, Me, Husband, Chiropractor, Therapist		
Medical Protocol	GammaKnife, CyberKnife		
	Tarceva		
Love	Husband, Grands, Close Friends, Community Present		
	Children, Extended Family, Community Past		
Joyful Activity	Laughing, Walking, Singing, Yoga, Biking		
	Playing, Dancing, Travelling, Canoeing		
Inner Conversation	Believing, Observing, Calming		
	Stilling, Deciding, Clearing		
Energy	Music, Goodwill, Qigong, Acupuncture		
	Jin Shin Jyutsu, Nature, Shaman		
Diet/ Supplement	Mushrooms, Decent diet		
	Vitamin D		

Will to live
Genes
Connection
Joyfulness
Strength
Experience
Spirit
Intelligence
Finances

Figure 5. My healing plan to this point

"Sarri, how many of your patients come into therapy with stacks of books and PowerPoints?" I ask at the end of the session. Gently she answers, "You know I'll always tell you the truth if you ask. No one." She pauses. "But maybe you were sent to the moon because you could describe the view."

How far in the future does this new view extend? While we wait for Dr. Mehta to arrive with the results from the long-anticipated, six-month post-CyberKnife scan, Thea tells the nurse in an apprehensive but insistent voice that "Nin's lungs are okay, they're okay." It turns out that she's right. Nothing in the irradiated area is growing, and there are no new tumors anywhere. Dr. Mehta is very pleased.

The nurse at the UW radiation oncology center gives me a thorough physical, trying to find something wrong in my brain, but she can't find anything. In fact she can't even see where the Gamma Knife procedure was done, much less something new.

"It's the most beautiful brain I've ever seen," she smiles. (I keep in mind she spends her days looking at scans of brain cancer patients, not yogis or monks, but I'm still grateful for her words.) She says I should continue with whatever I'm doing, and be thankful for my genes.

"You mean the genes that have given her cancer twice?" laughs Camilla, perhaps a little nervously, since she may share these genes.

"No, just the ones that have helped her survive it," the nurse laughs in reply.

Dr. Eaton is also excited: he hugs me twice. It's ironic that the formal information itself comes with so little fanfare; the one sentence of the radiology report says flatly, "Stable mass and three nodules are resolved."

I am ready to step over the line from patient to contributor. "How can I help other cancer patients?" I ask.

"That's a great lead-in," he replies. "As a matter of fact, Dr. Greg Holt, a pulmonologist from the Fred Hutchison Research Center is outside the door waiting for you. He'd like to use your blood for his research into a lung cancer vaccine."

Could my legacy be antibodies that could cure someone else? Wouldn't this be a great life purpose—bigger than anything I could have imagined? Wouldn't this make getting the cancer worthwhile?

Dr. Holt not only takes my blood, he listens to my story over a cup of coffee and takes the time to educate me further on the immune system and the biological processes underlying cancer. He asks me if he can show my presentation to the Tumor Vaccine Group at the University of Washington. Both of us are surprised when two hours have passed. It appears we've kept my son Eric waiting; my phone shows four missed calls from him.

"Did you check your e-mail?" Eric asks. He has sent me an ultrasound image. Of a little baby swimming in his mother's womb. The researchers might be addressing my life's grand purpose with the vaccine possibility, but I've now got a more immediate goal: to live to see the birth of a third grandchild.

Taking Reasonable Risks

There are no risk management strategies that prevent death, only those that may impact its timing. My view of the universe and my capacity for love are expanding. Why would I want to build a risk-free fence around my life when the view of the wide-open plains is so breathtaking? Because now I've got to stay alive until October.

In my next appointment, I ask Dr. Eaton how to avoid getting sick.

"All you can do is take reasonable risks," he replies.

When we have to jump back from the speeding bus that misses us by just inches on a narrow street, Kelly and I burst out laughing. A stock phrase that people use is, "You don't know that the cancer will get you. You could get hit by a bus." And now they were almost right. We are nearing the end of our maybe-the-last-vacation-before-Mom-dies trip and we've tried hard to minimize our risk—no exotic germs, long plane rides, or fatiguing sightseeing. Surely swimming poolside and sipping happy-hour margaritas are safe enough.

Or maybe not. I'm so busy worrying whether hot peppers plus Tarceva will set off the Tarceva Trots that I don't even consider Tarceva's propensity for eye irritation when I accept the complementary poolside facial. Whatever the woman put on my face starts to burn like a *habanero*, leaving me with two rings of fire around my eyes.

Surely singing is risk-free. But the next weekend, when I get ready to perform again with the Rural Characters, I forget that the 10-year-old makeup I apply to cover blisters from the facial might have accumulated its own pathogens in the years since it was last used.

That Monday, instead of hiking the nearby 200-foot bluff that falls precipitously to the beach (I'm sure-footed, really), we ride Kelly's motorcycle (the helmet's first-rate, I swear it) to the doctor to check out the sores on my cheeks and styes in my eyes. I'm worried about pinkeye with the grandkids coming to visit; the nurse is worried about shingles; and the doctor is worried about a staph infection, so she sends me home with an antibiotic.

Exercise is good for you, right? Thursday we hike the vineyards of Eastern Washington without considering the implications of 100-degree heat. When my back, leg, and feet muscles start to cramp that night, I'm concerned that it's an interaction between the antibiotic and the Tarceva. "Nothing so fancy," says the pharmacist, "it's probably just simple dehydration. Try Gatorade and a banana, and find somewhere cooler to hang out."

We head to the river but decide canoeing wouldn't be prudent because the rivers are overflowing with snowmelt, and capsizing would mean instant hypothermia. This proves to be smart—16 people are rescued from the river that day. But driving the four-mile dirt road into the canyon on our way to a quieter stream will prove not so smart when the road collects a piece of our transmission as a secret toll and two weeks later the car stops dead in the left lane of Interstate 5.

The little brook is beckoning when we arrive. Its riffles glisten, the shade is comforting, and the water patterns are beautiful—and so are the patterns on the rattlesnake two feet in front of me. But the snake and I agree that Death by Rattlesnake is not my destiny, at least not today, so I move to a spot in the stream where I can feel the water rush over me and visualize it cleansing me of any microscopic cancer that may still lurk in my bloodstream.

Kelly and I are exultant (another word for speeding) as we race to catch the 11:00 p.m. ferry. I only casually mention the soreness and new feeling of constriction in my throat when I run into Cathy, my primary care doc, at the local coffee hangout the next morning.

"Sore like a cold?"

"No, more like pressure, like not breathing."

"Stop the antibiotic immediately; you may be developing an allergic reaction."

When I get home and open my mail, I find the results of the lab work: I have a "rare staph infection." Rare? And they notify me by mail? Adrenalin starts running through my body as my web research indicates that some staph infections are deadly. I can't reach Cathy so I call the Seattle Cancer Care Alliance. Concerned, they tell me to come in immediately, and we rush across the ferry and through rush-hour traffic to get there.

En route, I get a call back from Cathy explaining that the note I had received was misleading: rare in this context means there was so little staph on my face that it was hard to find, and the staph that did exist was commonplace, not exotic.

"You were never in danger from staph," she says, "only from the antibiotic we gave you to cure it, the side effects from the drug we've given you for the cancer, and the poor choice of words we used that got you concerned."

In reviewing this crazy week, where was the greatest risk? The bus, the motorcycle ride, or the drive through rush-hour Seattle traffic? Was it the heat or the rattlesnake? My throat constricting, or the stress chemicals from worrying about it? Of the tools I used to avoid risk, which was the most powerful? The motorcycle helmet to protect me from an accident I might never have? The Tarceva to protect against a cancer that may no longer be there? Or the Gatorade to incorrect an imbalance I could definitely feel?

And where did the most healing take place? In the quiet of a rushing brook, or the laughter of friends around a campfire under a gibbous moon? In the exertion of a five-mile walk through vineyards, or carrying an infant on my chest on a beach at sunset? Or was it in the still of the night when I asked my body to clear the swelling from my eyes and throat, and restore its balance?

In every moment I face opportunities, and have to decide which ones to take and which to pass up, with little ability to truly assess either my risk or my thinking. I am learning to read outside signals and listen to internal ones, but I'm still a novice. But I know I'd rather open myself to life than to close myself off. I believe the greater risk for me lies not in not knowing, but in not growing. And I do know this: I have missed the opportunity to have the following said at my memorial service: "She faced down stage 4 cancer, a rattlesnake, and a speeding bus, but she was done in by a facial."

CHAPTER SEVEN

Diving Into
the Unknown

May–October, 2008

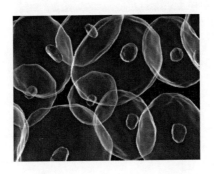

Kel and I always believed that we would both live to a productive and fulfilled age together and then die within hours, maybe days, no more than a couple of weeks of each other. I had an example of this in my own family when my grandfather succumbed to a heart attack only weeks before my grandmother expired of... lung cancer.

Frankly—and irrationally—this model has me worrying about Kel. He is so vigilant about every slight change in my health, but he doesn't pay as much attention to his own. I hesitantly broach the subject over dinner. The conversation goes about as well as you might expect—it stops abruptly. But so does Kel's overeating. He starts taking care of himself, and within weeks starts to transform in front of my eyes. The weight and fatigue of caregiving falls away. I marvel and delight in both his improved health and outlook.

I truly intend this time to be about him, for the focus to finally shift off me. But a little, niggling voice inside me asks if I want to restore his strength because intuitively I know that I'll need it again. I've had a delicious taste of survival, but within two weeks of our dinner conversation, I have another dream.

To: My wonderful support team
From: Diana
Date: July 25, 2008
Subject: The next walk

Dear wonderful support team,

Are you up for another leg on this amazing walk? We found out at the nine-month-post-CyberKnife scans that there is something new in my left lung. A small, 5mm speck just outside the area they treated with CyberKnife. While it is not definitively cancer, chances are good that it is, as it is located adjacent to the area of my original mass. But it is small. For perspective, the large mass I faced originally was 4cm x 3cm x 6cm and there were 3 more tumors in the brain, 2 in the right lung, and all the mediastinal nodes were involved. And we fought all that. We had Tarceva on our side along with Gamma Knife and CyberKnife, but my quality of life, well-being, and health are now so extraordinary by any measure that I know that we have all contributed our fair share toward this healing.

This time around the doctors don't want to do anything for at least 60 days and maybe 90. I will see my doctor in 30 but as long as I remain asymptomatic (which I am now—Kel and I walk 3–6 miles every day) he won't repeat the scans. So this leaves us in the enviable position of being able to fight this with daily exercise, energy treatments, meditation, and your healing prayers. I believe we can take care of this before my doctors have to bring in chemo or more radiation.

Medically I believe this is possible because I have learned that lung cancer is immunologic, meaning the immune system can recognize it and take care of it, to a point. But once it reaches a certain mass, the cancer starts to suppress the ability of the T-cells to recognize it. In other words, when the T-cell asks "are you a good cell or a bad cell?" the cancer starts to lie and becomes a wolf in sheep's clothing. Cancer cells also start sending excessive signals to their nuclei to reproduce. So in essence we have a communication problem. You and I know about communication problems. We solve them every day. And this one is still small.

Emotionally, Kelly and I are serene about this. Kelly describes it as "light." I had a dream a month before the test in which an alligator (the cancer) started to emerge from the vegetation and enter the world of people at the end of a driveway. A group of otters (the playful side of me that loves you all) scurried out and became sentries on a stone wall at the edge of the driveway. An owl (or maybe an eagle) swooped in and watched. Then two powerful Clydesdale horses (the Budweiser type) galloped in and blocked the entrance to the driveway in a show of strength, but they didn't confront the alligator either. The alligator was not aggressive to any of them. We were all on the top of a hill overlooking this scene (we have some perspective), and my friend Mary said, "Look! Nature is trying to resolve this herself." After watching the stand-off for a while we drove on past, and I said "I hope the alligator returns to where it belongs before 2:00, or else the medics, zookeepers, police, and firefighters waiting in the distance will think they've got to do something before the kids start walking home from school—and that won't be good for the alligator."

So I've already been made aware of the present scenario: instead of 2 o'clock, we have 2 months for "the alligator" to either go back to its habitat (the microscopic level where nobody cares) or transform into something that's healthy for my whole body. We know that this cancer has already transformed my life in most wondrous ways. So if you'd like to, please join me on top of that hill and send healing intentions. I'm thanking the alligator for bringing this to my attention, and the otters, owl/eagle, and horses for coming so quickly to my rescue. And I thank you as well.

I believe this will be OK. I am certainly way better than OK right now, and I know that together we are a mighty force. If I'm wrong, we'll try something else later.

Love,
Diana

Within a minute, my inbox starts to fill. "I'm joining the Clydesdales if you don't mind." Our friends, independent thinkers that they are, apparently don't want to stand on the hill passively observing. By email this morning they are not only closing ranks on the alligator, they are transforming themselves into animal spirits. The line between my inner world and my daily life is becoming more porous. Whether friends are near or far, they're willing to pass without hesitation through the portal of my imagination and become active agents.

But now that we are all nicely lining this driveway, what precisely are we doing? How exactly is "nature going to take care of it?" Is it enough to just wait here, in solidarity? Will the alligator slink off on its own, happy to return to its native habitat, or is there something I'm supposed to do to encourage its retreat?

Acupuncture: Balancing the Energy Flow

It's a very different world from the Seattle Cancer Care Alliance. Tim Batiste's office is in a comfortable old clapboard house in downtown Langley instead of a large hospital in Seattle. There are no nurses or staff. I hear Tim's laughter through the thin walls of his waiting room before I meet him. A second-generation acupuncturist, unusual in our country for a non-Chinese, he exudes ease, warmth, and good humor as he listens to me recount my medical history. But he's most interested in my spirit's history—my joy at having made it this far, my continued fear for the future, my willingness to entertain a connection to forces larger than myself—that he somehow elicits without directly probing.

He starts with a typical first-time treatment for patients who have undergone chemo or radiation. Its goal is to rid the body of toxins and the heart of old emotions—like an exorcism. As I lie on the table for 20 minutes with needles draining away the negative energy, I have a meditation of being swept down class-four rapids, tossed between the boulders of my parents, falling over the rocks of cancer, until I can finally get onshore onto a beach where I am rapidly sorting bad petals from good. When Tim tells me the treatment is called *Seven Dragons on Seven Demons*, my eyes open at its ability to surface my own demons.

So as Tim continues the treatment, I ask what he is doing.

"I'm strengthening your liver, your recycling center."

Good, I'm ready to take the energy I've spent on these memories and put it to better use.

"I'm strengthening the point called "the Gate between Heaven and Earth;" it keeps you grounded in living."

Lastly Tim boosts my energy with specific points on meridians that he calls my foundational issues: my heart beats strongly but the layer designed to protect it needs strengthening.

The names of the treatments are poetic instead of the numbers associated with a clinical trial. The wall charts of the meridians superimposed on the body are different from the anatomical drawings in Dr. Eaton's textbooks. Cognitively, I'm already so deep in dissonance that a little more is hardly noticeable. Emotionally, I'm still surprised by the force of the meditation. Physically, the energy sensations aren't that strong; it takes a day before I realize my body is somehow just flowing better. But intuitively, I like Tim. I want him on my team. He doesn't think I'm in crisis so I agree to come back only monthly.

When I return for my July appointment and tell Tim about the recurrence on my scans, he is surprised. When I share the alligator dream, he listens wide-eyed but intently. He starts his treatment with the point "Utmost Source" to stimulate my ability to tap into the energy source without limits.

"A cancer diagnosis is just the starting point, Diana. Our healing potential is infinite if we can tap into the source," he says encouragingly.

And then he opens up a point called "Windows of the Sky" which he uses only when someone is clear and directed and knows life is moving in the right direction. It is not a point he typically uses with someone who has just received a cancer diagnosis or evidence of a recurrence because clarity at that moment can simply be too devastating. But my dream gives him confidence that I am truly looking for insight, that I have the strength to handle whatever that insight decrees, and that I have dream guides to help me along the way. So he intuits that I will need a clean view of the upcoming healing path.

He finishes with the heart protector, the "Heavenly Spring." "Fire is your constitutional element," he explains, "and when we direct the energy into who you are everything else comes into alignment."

And who I am in this moment is someone with the fire to get well. The fewer tools Dr. Eaton has in his back pocket, the more I need in mine. I am grateful for the help that Tim, Sarri and Jill continue to give me during our appointments but seeing them monthly, bi-weekly or even weekly is simply not enough. I want to try to keep my body tuned to a constant state of wellness. We've been trying to do this already with diet, exercise, and the Joy Protocol. What more can we try? Or is it something less?

Reiki: Channeling Universal Energy

Total immersion has long been the preferred way to learn a language, which is why Kelly says that five years of High School Spanish prepared him for nothing more than ordering off the drive-up menu at Taco Bell, and why I learned French in two weeks when that was the only language I could use to speak to the blond-haired, blue-eyed, Norwegian boy who sat next to me in a Swiss classroom.

"You can't become totally immersed in something if you're already immersed in something else," Kel says. "Now I understand why so many meditative traditions emphasize emptiness. You've got to drain everything else away in order to pave the way for infinite possibility."

So we've decided what we have to do with this new cancer growth.

"Total immersion. Climb the ladder to the high board, and dive into an empty pool," Kel says. "Symbolically, of course."

Kel immediately signs up for a Reiki workshop. Reiki is another hands-on healing method from Japan that Kel has been reading about. The idea of learning about this appeals to him; attending a workshop does not. But he goes.

That evening when he gives me a treatment, Kelly's palms are on fire. So what happened to him in that workshop? Reiki is about a fundamental transformation of some kind that allows the practitioner to facilitate the flow of life-energy, and it's entirely up to the person being treated to draw the energy in and use it in whatever way is most useful. Does it really work that way?

"Maybe. Maybe not," says Kel. But he's no longer so convinced that just because something can't be measured doesn't mean it doesn't exist, that just because it can't be proven or repeated doesn't mean it didn't happen. "On the other hand," he counters, "just because it *did* happen and can't be explained doesn't mean the fairies did it; we want to be open-minded, not empty-headed. Then again, maybe the fairies did do it," Kel suggests over breakfast, with only the hint of a grin.

When Thea turned four, she was really into "Cats," the musical. When next-door-nephew John asked her why Mr. Mistoffelees was magical, as the song says, Thea replied: "Well, I don't know exactly why he's magical because the man who made him up is dead, so we can't ask him. But in the song Mr. Mistoffelees pulls seven kittens right out of a hat, so I think that's pretty magical, don't you? So that's my theory right now," she answers (yes, she said "theory," or rather "pheory," since she still had a lisp.) "But if you ask me later, I might think something different."

That works for Kel and me. At this particular point about the only conviction we have left is that conviction itself is overrated. Anything—no matter how impossible or improbable—is fair game in the pursuit of health and happiness. For both of us.

Qigong: Making Our Own Medicine

After the Reiki workshop, Kel's hands are always "on." He gives me treatments whenever he can: as simply as laying his hand on my lung when we're out at the movies, as sensitively as balancing my whole body on our massage table at home, and as magically as lying in the middle of Yosemite Valley and feeling the energy rush down the granite face of El Capitan, across the Merced River, through my body, and up Glacier Point.

But I want a way to get 24 x 7 healing without always asking Kel or retreating to a corner to do my visualizations or a traditional Qigong practice. I haven't been taught how to do this in class but it simply isn't practical for me to be waving my arms everywhere I go. People would stare, Kel would get kicked in bed, and Thea would worry. I've been working on a way to help my fellow cancer survivors access Qigong in less than five minutes and now I'm trying it myself so I can extend my healing to every waking moment. So whether I'm still or active, prone or upright, by myself or in the company of others, eyes open or closed, I bring in healing energy and circulate it through my body. I "run loops," a combination of the imagery that worked so well for me and the Yi Ren Qigong practice I've learned in class.[74] I run the loops in my mind but I feel the energy sensations in my body. I had purposely not guided my meditations in the healing glen but this time I experiment with setting an intention for the meditation before I start it. The energy flows on its own from there.

The first loop, called the *"Small Universe"* in class, is a circle of energy that moves up the back and down the front of my torso. I intend for it to reinforce all the systems of my body, strengthening them so they can support the tremendous self-healing effort. Sometimes I just feel Qi or energy tingling through my body, other times I visualize water carrying out the dead cells and recharging my batteries.

I use the second loop, the *"Large Universe,"* to connect to power sources outside of myself, water from deep in the earth, light from the sun. The loop carries water up the front of the body, from my toes to my upstretched fingers, to clear all the communication channels between the cells. Down the back of my body, it brings light to recognize the tumor and heat to burn it out.

The third loop, called the *"Extraordinary Universe,"* aims to boost the power of the endocrine and immune system and reverse the damage caused by stress chemicals. I focus my intention on igniting the restorative power of the bone marrow—my very own bone marrow transplant. As the energy moves up the inside of my spinal cord, I pause it at my adrenal glands to clear the stress. As it moves up my neck, over my ear and into the center of my head, I tell the hypothalamus, guardian of the body, to relax and stop sending stress signals. As the energy moves down the front I watch it ignite the protective power of the immune system, in the sinus, thyroid, thymus, and spleen.

Now, really, can I do this? That's easy: yes. I feel the Qi at work in my body. It's not only a sensation of a current, a tingling, but it's a force capable of moving on its own. Am I achieving the inner alchemy I hope for? That I won't know for a while. But at minimum, the exercise is soothing, calming, yet energizing. Do I have any real understanding of how that might possibly work? No, but I'm OK with mystery these days, and I take some consolation in research done on pianists, athletes and performers that show their skills improving through visualization.

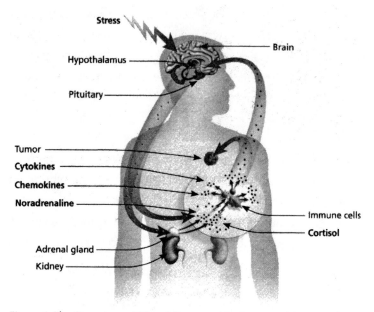

Figure 6. The Stress Loop. When I first saw this diagram of the stress loop in Dr. Servan-Shreiber's book *Anticancer*,[75] I was interested to note that the "Extraordinary Universe" loop follows the reverse path of the stress loop.

So I add a fourth loop over my lung, a swirling vortex the size of a campaign button, which I think of as my personal chemo port to the energies of the universe. But what's the best source of energy to plug into? It's natural to consider sun, water, and, ground. It's easy to feel the love that flushes my body as I snuggle with my grandchildren. It's possible to feel the power of sequoia, redwood, and fir, as their sap pumps hundreds of feet into the air (yes, I am confessing to being a tree-hugger). It's astonishing and delightful to be close enough to an apple tree in 90-degree heat to feel the cool of its respiration. It's effortless to feel the communion between friends as salmon filets grill on the deck, or foil-wrapped trout cooks over the campfire. But it's more of a challenge when driving through some parts of Interstate 5 to imagine that anything in this mass of asphalt and signage could be beneficial to my health. So on this ride home to the ferry I focus on the motion of the tires revolving under us, giving energy to my body's healing just as they give energy back to the battery of our Prius.

I am present. Kel is present. We are breaking through to a level of connection with our universe we have never experienced; we are plugging into the master grid, and we are happy. And it is a time of breakthroughs for our children as well.

Marin Alsop made history as the first woman to lead a major U.S. orchestra. Director of the Cabrillo Music Festival since 1992—a festival that has garnered the coveted ASCAP award for Adventurous Programming in Contemporary Music every year she's been there—she is the person who the world's great living composers turn to in order to bring their music alive with all the passion, fire, nuance, and power it deserves. Alsop herself has a grueling schedule, one that doesn't end when she retires to a hotel room in a distant city. Scores from countless composers and publishers await her review long into the night.

For the opening night of this year's Cabrillo Festival, she has selected four pieces: one of these she commissioned herself, and another is by our 28-year-old son, Eric. "Darkness Made Visible" was one of those unsolicited scores that somehow made it to her in one of those hotel rooms (as she tells the audience in the pre-opening gala), and she" just liked it." The odds of Eric's work being on this program are even more outrageous than the odds that his mother would be there to watch it.

☉ ☉ ☉

A few weeks later, elbows down, hands clenched by his armpits, an ecstatic smile on his face, 31-year-old Isaac starts jumping up and down on the sidewalk between Café de la Presse and a parking garage in San Francisco. Camilla catches the fever and starts jumping, too, elbows and hands matching Isaac's, igniting Thea, whose leaps from her orange crocs nearly cause her to drop her orange stuffed parrot. Isaac has just heard that he has won the prestigious Betty Bowen award from the Seattle Art Museum. His work will be displayed there for a year. Is breaking through the limits of what we once thought impossible contagious? For our family right now, exhilaration seems to be.

To: My wonderful support team
From: Diana
Date: September 5, 2008
Subject: We did it!

Dear amazing team,

We got the results of my latest CT today and there is no growth. The speck *is* in check.

Let's not even pretend we know why. But know that I am elated and so very grateful to you, my wonderful family and friends, who have held me in your hearts for 28 months (let's hear that again, 28! a far cry from the 3–12 it could have been). You are a mighty force.

Love,
Diana

Standing in my mother's kitchen drying the last dishes from a late-night dinner, we get a rushed call from Eric. After six weeks of hospitalization for placenta previa, Kylie needs an emergency C-section. The surgical procedure she believes best is a tricky one. Her doctor, an hour away on a family vacation, knows how to do it. His partner, overbearing and on call, does not. He insists that both her life and the baby's are in jeopardy if Kylie doesn't immediately consent to a different type of surgery. Kylie considers this, and refuses. She is waiting for her own doctor, who is by this time speeding to the hospital.

Before Kel even gets off the phone I'm busy trying to book the next flight out of three different airports, but there is nothing available before 6:00 am. We retreat upstairs where I slide down the edge of the bed onto the floor and try to do what others have done for me: beam light, send healing energy, pray. Sitting there in the dark teaches me something else about caregiving. It *does* take courage to listen to your body's guidance over your doctor's, but it takes just as much courage from those who love you—especially when they fear your life is on the line. Eric trusts Kylie. That's all that really matters.

Our second grandson safely breaks through at 11:22 that night, on October 18th, with the help of both surgeons who operated together. When we arrive the next morning, Kylie wakes up and smiles at me.

"Do you remember that meditation you had during Gamma Knife and how there were three grandchildren in it? Meet Aidan."

Three safe and happily fall asleep, I sing softly as I first hold him in my arms.

CHAPTER EIGHT

The Space Between, or The Complexity of Connection

November, 2008–February, 2009

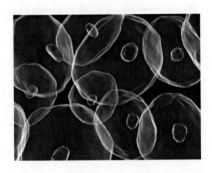

Dr. William Parks is Director of the Center for Lung Biology at the University of Washington. Five minutes before we're to meet, I download my first app on my new iPhone: a voice recorder. If this conversation goes as I hope, I know I won't understand half the words being used.

We're meeting at Daniel's Broiler, the place in Seattle where aerospace engineers, software wizards, and biotech researchers go for business lunches. Deals are struck, ideas hatched, and visions entertained, but even by Daniel's Broiler standards I think we might venture into some new territory. I want to know if any of my imagery could be of any use to the research community. A big part of me can't believe I'm about to have this conversation, but after we quickly order, I nervously pull out a printed version of my "Stage IV Lung Cancer from the Inside" Powerpoint, press the big red "record" button on my iPhone and hope it works.

"Since I was first diagnosed I have had visualizations of inner healers working to remove the cancer. I thought at first that they were simply a unique language my mind and my body had come up with to talk to each other during this fight, but as I've learned more about the actual biological processes in my body, I'm increasingly struck by how similar the images seem to what's really going on at a medical level. Recently I went back through my journal to find the dates of these meditations and then reviewed all of my CT reports. The progression of the images correlates *in every case* with my clinical results. Would you be willing to see if I've correctly understood the biology, and help me fill in some gaps?"

I can almost watch Bill's mind shift as he readies himself to follow me down a metaphor-strewn path. I love world-class scientists who are open to trying on even the strangest-sounding new ideas to advance their research.

"You know that there is precedence for scientists using their own dreams to help them solve a puzzle in their research," Bill says, "The structure of the benzene ring was discovered that way, and there are other examples in the literature. So yes, by all means, continue."

Knowing that I'm talking with a scientist, I explain the methodology I've used to create the PowerPoint I'm going to show him. I've searched Google for images that most closely resemble my memory of what each meditation looked like. Also, on each slide I've included the correlation of my clinical results and my hypotheses about what the actual disease or immunological process might have been.

I start with April 25, 2006 and the image of Lung Woman with a giant boulder on her chest, then describe my original tumor burden. I tell him about the women who were symbols for my different organ systems, and how they beamed light at me for a week, after which one of the lesions was gone (on May 12). I show him an image of water pouring through my brain and tell him how my current scans show that all the post-Gamma Knife scarring in my brain is gone.

"I think that imagery of light and water are very common in our collective unconsciousness, so I don't think they correlate to a specific biological process, although I do know there is research on using light therapy for cancer," I say. Bill is clearly still working to wrap his mind around what I'm saying.

I show him the pictures of how Tarceva works—how its goal is to plug up a specific receptor on the cell, and how similar that is to my visualizations of dancers stomping on bubble wrap (see figure 7). He can't help but smile at the toe-shoe picture.

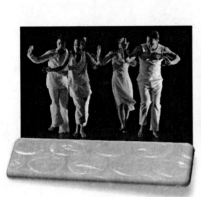 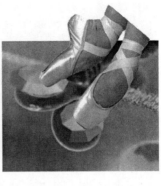

Figure 7. The dance images on the left (from Tandy Beal's *Here After Here*) represent the jumping, stomping, and sliding the inner dancers do in order to pop the "bubble wrap" of the cell. The image on the right is from a video on the Genentech website. It represents Tarceva as a gold disk plugging up the red EGFR/HER-1 receptor (I added the toe shoes).

"Even I laughed at my own imagination, but after these meditations, my May 26, 2006 CT showed the tumor had shrunk in half." This gets his attention.

"In June of 2006 the stomping in my visualizations released bubbles that quickly filled the space where the dancers were working," I continue. "When I saw a picture of cancer cells dying on an airport magazine stand, I was struck by how familiar the image was." (See figure 8.)

"Yes, the bubbles, as you call them, of a dying cell's membrane are called blebs," Bill explains.

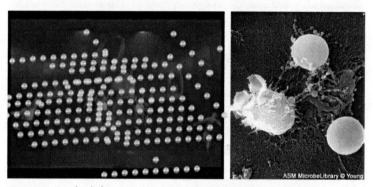

Figure 8. On the left is my representation of the bubbles that were released as the dancers continued to pop bubble wrap. On the right is an image of apoptosis, cell death, I found on the UW Tumor Vaccine Group website before giving blood for vaccine research.[76]

I tell Bill how on June 2, circus acrobats inserted vaulting poles into my lungs to help the bubbles evacuate the area more efficiently (see figure 9a). Bill is clearly intrigued by the poles. He says, "To fight cancer you need the help of a specific type of immune cell that can recognize the tumor cell is different from a healthy cell, sound an alert, and guide in killer T-cells to do the nasty job of killing the cell. What's fascinating is that there are some beautiful photographs of this process, that, while not as perfect as your imagery here, show that these immune cells attach themselves to cable-like structures and ride in together to the rescue." (See figure 9b.)

I'm too flabbergasted to say anything for a moment (and even more so when I see the actual picture—above—that Bill e-mails after our conversation). "Is this how my tumor shrank in half again on the June 23rd CT scan?" I wonder out loud. "The rest of that summer the meditations were all about water. As I stand in a river the nutrients I need enter my shoulder blades, the water flows down my chest destroying the cancer, and the byproducts emerge from my navel in a constant downriver flow."

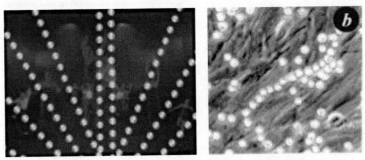

Figure 9. On the left is my image of the poles. The image on the right is a picture by Carol de la Motte of the Cleveland Clinic of immune cells, called monocyte/macrophages, riding in to the tumor on an express-bus-like cable, called hyaluronan (HA).[77] HA is made of carbohydrates in the extracellular matrix. Research shows that exercise (like the walking I was doing at the time of this meditation) increases the number of monocyte/macrophages available to fight a tumor.[78]

Bill interjects, "Right. That's interstitial fluid, which constantly flows from the vasculature, through our tissues, and into the lymphatic system. The whole immune system takes advantage of this riverworks system to do its job."

"The next image was straightforward," I continue. "On November 22 I had a dream about the healer massaging the lymph nodes in my mediastinum, the area in my chest between my lungs. My December 13 CT revealed that the mediastinal lymph nodes were free of cancer. This was the first time I began to seriously consider the synchronicity of my meditative images with my clinical results."

Bill nods. He's with me now.

"The next series of images occurred in mid-December 2006, about 9 months after my diagnosis. Instead of the tumor repeatedly shrinking in half on every CT, the tumor mass stabilized at 2.0 x 1.0 cm. The dancers didn't have much space left and resorted to jumping up and down like Balkan folk dancers in mountainous country where flat land is scarce. The surface of what they were stomping on changed as well. Instead of popping bubble wrap, they were now trying to chip away on a lava-like structure to no avail. Compared to the earlier cancer cells that would immediately pop when stomped, this stuff was dense and hard. I don't know whether it was scar tissue, or some other type of cell that I was dealing with."

"Yes, the tumor encases itself in scar tissue that is very durable," says Bill, jumping back in. "The components of scar connective tissue are mostly collagen. Leather is collagen. Scar tissue also contains elastin, the material that makes your skin return to its original shape when stretched. It's so durable that you take the elastin you're born with to the grave. So I agree that beating down this lava would take a long time." (See figure 10.)

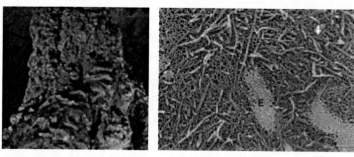

Figure 10. On the left is a lava spire I found on Google that most closely resembled my memory of the lava in my meditation. The figure on the right is scar tissue made up of collagen and elastin (E) fibers. Collagen is derived from the Greek word *kolla* meaning glue.[79]

Turning the page, I go on: "The image I particularly wanted to show you was when the central healer finds a new kind of cell with many tentacles like the roots of a tree. She thinks she will never be able to identify the edges of all of those little tentacles well enough to extract them without breaking off a piece that could cause damage later. But she comes up with a solution: she injects pink fluid into the cell with a syringe, as if she was filling a crumpled rubber glove with fluid, and the glove expands to reveal its true shape and boundaries." (See figure 11.)

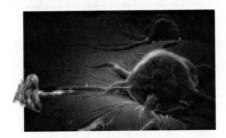

Figure 11. This image represents the difficulties the healer has in trying to extract a multi-tentacled stem cell without leaving anything behind.

"You mean something inside the cell then reveals these tentacles so we can see them more easily?" Bill asks.

"Yes, the image made me believe that therapies that target only the outside receptors, like many of the current anti-cancer drugs, won't be enough to cure cancer. To fully understand the cancer, you have to come from the inside out, not just the outside in.'"

Considering this, Bill says, "Well, the first thing that comes to my mind are tumor antigens. Many academic groups, like Dr. Nora Disis's lab at the University of Washington, and pharmaceutical companies are trying to exploit tumor antigens to develop tumor vaccines to stimulate immune cells to kill the cancer cells."

"Like my image of the syringe?"

He nods.

"At the end of this imagery, the healer turned the glove-like cell inside out so that it stood up like a tree and then blasted it. This image took place in February 28, 2007. Dr. Greg Holt from Dr. Disis's lab told me it takes 4–5 months to go from stem cell to a tumor that's visible on a CT. Sure enough, my August 24, 2007 scan showed there was new growth, and I used the imagery to guide me in choosing a blast-like radiation treatment called CyberKnife."

"The mass is still there today? What are you visualizing now?" Bill asks.

"Yes, it's still there but hasn't grown in five months. I've been thinking about how a successful tumor mass sends its tentacles between healthy cells and robs them of resources.

Well, what are these healthy cells doing? Are they inadvertently colluding with the cancer cells? Or is their attention diverted elsewhere? Now I've been wondering if there's some gunk, like some fortified sludge, between the cells that the cancer cells thrive in?"

"There is. Actually I'm the president of the American Society for Gunk," he says wryly.

We both laugh.

"Is there a more formal name for it?" I ask.

"The extracellular matrix is probably the gunk you're talking about. It *does* lie between every cell. Very few cells touch membrane to membrane." (See figure 12.)

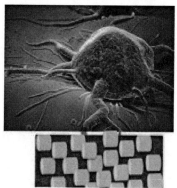
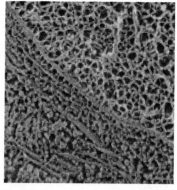

Figure 12. The left-hand image shows the cancer cell sending its roots between the cells, either creating or growing in a "gunky" environment between the cells. On the right is an image of a cell (upper right), the cell membrane (the diagonal line) and the actual extracellular matrix (lower left), which is rich in carbohydrates and other elements. The matrix can get clogged with versican, creating an inflammatory environment that helps the cancer metastasize throughout the body.[80]

Completely incredulous that I have found this particular expert just when I'm trying to work through this specific visualization, I say, "So the solution to the gunk was a response by the healthy cells: they needed to be active, stronger, to 'loosen up' so they could break free of the hold of the gunk, allowing nourishment to come in and clean water to clear out the bad soil." Bill smiles in confirmation. In January, Bill and I will make a correlation between the gunk and a protein called versican. Versican is normally found in small amounts in healthy lung tissue, but in January 2009, scientists from the University of California at San Diego found it in large amounts in aggressive lung tumors.[81] Advanced cancer cells commandeer components from the immune system to generate an inflammatory microenvironment—gunk?—that the cancer uses as a highway to grow and metastasize.

"So when are you going to publish this?" he asks. "Personally, the data in my experiments is pretty dry and empirical compared to this kind of thinking, but there is so much we don't understand about nature. We don't understand how our own body works, how our central nervous system and our brain interact. We do know that the brain sends out feelers to every part of our body in a way that we don't yet understand. Your images might be related to that. They open a door that helps me think out the box."

Bill leafs quickly back through the presentation. "I like the guy bringing in the poles with the bubbles. When I get back to my office, I'll send you the paper on this," he says thumping the image for emphasis. And then he pauses. "And this alligator head, it's just the snout?"

I nod.

With obvious empathy he says, "That can't be a good image."

"No, it's terrifying." And suddenly we're not a researcher and a patient, but fellow human beings.

A week later, Bill asks if he can show my presentation to a friend newly-diagnosed with cancer. I had considered these images to be a reflection of the status of the cancer within my body communicated in a private language. Could it be possible to use images of healthy cells and molecular processes as a dynamic, proactive instruction set for others?

⊙ ⊙ ⊙

After my December scans still show no growth on the small spot found on July's CT, or anywhere else, we learn about another possibility—that the lack of growth might not be the result of our prodigious efforts but simply a reflection of the new spot not having been cancer in the first place. Dr. Holt tells us about "Very small (3–5 millimeter) well-defined nodules often seen on CT examinations of the chest. These nodules have commonly been referred to as 'ditzels,' possibly because of the lack of a better term."[82] His comment reminds me of looking spellbound at the lungs in the *Bodies* exhibit that was touring the nation. The smokers' lungs were black, and the miners' lungs were a horrifying coal-black, but even the healthy lungs were speckled, like sidewalks with ground-in chewing gum.

According to a study published in 2010, some of these spots show up on CT scans. In fact, ¼ of the spots that show up on CTs turn out not to be cancer. So what do doctors do about this? According to Lee F. Rogers, MD, Editor in Chief of the *American Journal of Roentgenology*: "At times, the hardest thing to do with small findings is nothing—that is, to dismiss the finding as irrelevant and unimportant. A good diagnostician is one who is willing to overlook, or has the ability to dismiss, such ditzels with certainty and not request further examinations or follow-up studies... It is a matter of judgment, and some of us are better at this than others."[83]

So is the spot cancer or a ditzel? Given how close the spot is to the original mass, Dr. Eaton believes it is cancer. In the absence of growth, however, he is willing to continue the wait-and-see approach.

Resonating: The Power of Our Social Network

I've brought Thea and Camilla with me to a morning performance of the Seattle Symphony. As the first chord in the Britten piece rushes over us, we feel like the guy in the commercial whose hair is blasted straight back by the sound coming from his home entertainment system. Thea's delight is infectious. She recognizes the trumpet's theme from a YouTube clip we watched the night before, and starts jumping up and down in her seat, like a horse ready to gallop. I move her quickly to my lap before the ushers notice. Camilla and I feel the urge as well, although we manage to control ourselves.

After the concert, I drive over to a weekend Qigong seminar with Dr. Sun—Kel's first and my third. My focus shifts from sound waves boldly emanating from an orchestra to energy waves radiating more subtly from other people. We begin an exercise aimed at clearing energy in the stomach and pancreas meridians, but energy isn't moving up and transforming as it usually does in my body. Instead it remains stuck, heavy, and persists through lunch.

During the Q&A after lunch, I ask Dr. Sun, "I don't have any trouble with my stomach or pancreas, so why is this so difficult for me? And why do I feel so sad?"

"I think you are picking up energy from the people around you, Diana," reflects Dr. Sun. "Even cells can show the 'emotions' of ill-health if you introduce toxins into a petri dish. But if you replace the environment, the cell rebounds with astonishing resilience. You have a tremendous ability to absorb the grief, sorrow, and frustration of others. It is an amazing quality, but it comes at too great a cost to your body. When you see this kind of energy coming towards you, you have to stop it at the entry point. Go 'click' in your mind and either don't take it in, release it as soon as you discover it, or transform it. And this is the wonderful thing: our conscious minds can override the emotion. You can decide."

Yesterday I had seen a fellow lung cancer survivor in Dr. Eaton's waiting room, and I was dismayed by the toll the cancer was taking. Before we could talk, the nurse rushed me into the examining room to take my blood pressure. 150. I'm normally 120.

"Were you aware of the effect on your body of feeling upset?" asks Sarri later.

"No." At the time my body felt normal, like everything was under control. Perhaps, despite what Dr. Sun says, the price of having our talented mirror neurons is that our bodies can't help but feel each other's pain.

And pain is everywhere in our family now. Tom and Susan postponed a decision to divorce when I was first diagnosed so the family wouldn't suffer two blows at once. But now that time has come. We love them both, we understand their needs, and we support their decision, but that doesn't take away the sense of loss we all feel, having loved them as a family for more than 35 years. The Family Compound that was a source of such joy during the summer of 2006 is now full of sorrow. Kel's parents, who rushed to our support during the Love-In, rush back again, but this time there's no Jin Shin or Rural Characters to lighten the moments, no common purpose to unite us.

This is what comes from surviving, of being part of a family, connected to each other in ways we don't need to express with words. At least that's the way it is for me. I have spent the last three years opening up every pore and receptor I have to life and to others.

I have dismantled the protective barriers that allow us to sit on a subway without reaching out to ease another's suffering. I have turned up my inner receiver, and when I borrow Tom's truck one afternoon, I feel his grief all around me as clearly as if it was being broadcast on AM radio. I cry. When I listen to Susan's anger, all I can manage is to hold her in light, trying to keep my own candle from being blown out by the gale.

I am lousy at holding emotion at the entry point. There is no button to "click" in sight. And I am not alone. Ronald and Jan Glaser from Ohio State University's College of Medicine will demonstrate in 2012 that mirror neurons do contribute to social contagion. When love is in a room, we all get a hit of the dopamine rush but we can "catch" pain just as easily. Our mirror neurons mimic, our bodies feel, and then we share those feelings and in the process amplify them. The result can be distressing: our immune response is weakened by negative, hostile, contemptuous, or simply unhappy behavior. Humans are as impacted by our families as a cell is affected by the extracellular matrix and, as it turns out, a gene by the epigene. You can't heal the one without considering the many.

Epigenetics: The Power of Our Cell's Environment

The next day in class, Dr. Sun discusses Chinese medicine's view of the inter-relationships between the organs of the body and the meridians, including the paired meridians of the lung and large intestine. He explains how an imbalance in one of the meridians can stress the other—an explanation perhaps for my getting both colon and lung cancer. He then talks about the protective power of the reproductive/lymphatic system, which after a hysterectomy, is now compromised.[84]

Dr. Sun also talks about how Qigong works on the cellular level. He believes it corrects problems with our epigenetic layer. Did I hear that right? Epigenetics, the study of how genes can be turned on or off by factors other than your genetic code, like in my "goo" meditation? Epigenetics and Qigong? Leading-edge scientific theory and ancient Chinese medicine. How would *that* work?

Epigenetics is complex because researchers suspect that many things impact this layer: what we eat and don't eat, what we do and don't do, what toxins we're exposed to—even at levels far below current safety standards. In 2010 Stephen Rappaport, Professor of Environmental Health at UC Berkley will write in *Science Magazine* that "70–90% of disease risks are probably due to differences in environment."[85] Not genes.

Despite the complexity, there's hope in this: we are not just victims of our genetic code. What can change for the worse can possibly change for the better. "Unknown" is a word scientists actually use when talking about epigenetics, making me feel quite at home. The article "Medicine's new epicenter? Epigenetics" in *Cure* magazine I had read in March had in fact concluded with: "It is as if scientists have suddenly been handed the keys to a sports car they never knew existed, with no idea where the road trip will take them."[86]

Dr. Sun suggests that Qigong can help with the navigation. "For many health concerns, the underlying DNA sequence of the genes in the body doesn't change. Instead, non-genetic factors like diet, toxins, and exercise cause the genes to behave or express themselves differently. Our Qigong practice can help us recognize which factors contribute to healing and increase our quality of life; and which factors trigger our genes into unhealthy directions," he explains.

Dr. Sun believes western medicine excels at emergency treatments such as traumatic physical injuries, crisis care, and life-or-death situations. "To borrow from the language of computer science, modern western medicine has focused on the care and management of the body's 'hardware.' On the other hand, Qi cultivation excels at treating non-crisis illness, such as chronic pain, type 2 diabetes, arthritis, insomnia, chronic fatigue syndrome, fibromyalgia, and others."

"But how does this happen?" a student asks.

"The Qi pathway system is an interface between the physical body's hardware and the body's 'software'—the mind, consciousness, memories, emotions, and intelligence of the body," Dr. Sun continues. "It's like an energetic operating system in the body for the physiological, emotional, and psychological applications running in the body in our daily lives."

Then he adds that this operating system can get bugs in it. Sometimes, like with our computers, some sleep is all we need to "reboot." If that's not enough, he assures us that Qigong can help us go back to the source code and re-install it.

So that night I'm in bed wondering exactly *how* do I go back to the source code for re-installation? Did I miss something Dr. Sun said? Did my focus wander just at the critical moment? Was there a six-disc pack with an "Install Me" file that I forgot to pick up at the end of class? How do I turn this metaphor into molecule?

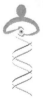

Mary, my wise friend in the alligator dream, is crying. I follow her to a beautiful conference center with flowers, blooming trees, and fountains; crowds of people are streaming into it. Now I can't find Mary, so I decide to go in and save her a spot. There are two lectures about to start: 'Surviving Relationships in the 21st Century,' and 'Sustainable Living.' I think she is going into 'Surviving Relationships' so I look for her there. A small intimate group starts asking me questions and laughs as I entertain them with stories about getting rid of my dog.

> *But I realize this is not where Mary was heading. As I leave*
> *for the other lecture, which is in a much larger hall, I see*
> *Mary in the plaza. She hasn't even had time to brush her hair.*
> *'Mary, why are you crying?' I ask…*

…and I wake up. No, don't wake up now! Mary is the one who had said, "Nature is taking care of it," in the alligator dream, so I urgently want to return to the dream and find out why she's crying. Sleep doesn't come, but in that twilight state my body starts to talk to me in a new way. Its energy moves slowly from its deepest parts to concentrate within an organ. I observe where my body is generating heat, and my attention walks over to warm itself by the fire. I just focus on the Qi, without analysis or interpretation. My cells know more about their inner workings than I ever will. My role here is simply to give my love and attention to whichever organ requests it, so I slip into a Qigong meditation where my body communicates not through visual imagery but through sensation.

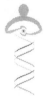 *I feel my heart glowing. It feels warm, and the energy under my hands pops like red-hot lava bubbling in the crater of a volcano. Now I'm aware of the energy shifting to my brain. It tingles. I notice that it's following the Qigong pathway that we have just learned. It moves over every corner of my brain like a river, searching out corrupt code and running waves of new self-healing code from front to back.*

Then I feel the sensation move to my kidneys, where the energy feels both warm and sparkling, like electricity. My kidneys are pulsing loudly, strongly, and my attention stays with them for a few minutes until they settle down.

Then the energy moves to my liver.

Until now the meditation has been becoming aware of my energy-body in a new way. But apparently my body recognizes that I'm only just learning this language, so it switches back to our mother tongue, visualization, and (just to be sure I'm following the conversation correctly) returns full circle to the organs-as-people imagery we used together after I was first diagnosed.

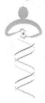

My liver is a young, vigorous man with Dr. Sun's build. He is running a marathon, maybe multiple marathons. He says, 'I'm just fine, don't worry' and indeed, he looks like he can go forever.

But I say to him 'I know you have the strength, but nevertheless we will find a way for you to get some rest. Thank you for your efforts.' He gives me a chipper salute as he runs off, knees high, carrying his baton.

My hands return to my heart, where my Heart Woman looks vibrantly healthy. I ask her, 'What's happening with Left Lung Woman?' and then, as if in answer to my question, she appears—a stooped, pock-faced crone. She has been through a lot. But I realize that she knows how to rewind the spool of time, and right before my eyes she transforms to my younger self, long brown hair, dancer body, and all.

Although I'm awestruck by this conversation, I have enough presence of mind to ask, 'Can I see Right Lung Woman?'

She already looks like me at my current age, and seems well enough, but when I think, 'Let's give her some added vitality,' she becomes even younger. The three women— the Goddess, Left Lung Woman, and Right Lung Woman—then stand on top of my chest, glowing, like the scene in Star Wars when the original Jedi masters return to their true selves, uncorrupted and fully aligned with the Force.

This is fun, let's keep going. What's going on in my brain? Brain Woman expands to fit the entire cranial cavity. This seems like a good sign.

And what about my kidneys? In the ship that is my body they are crammed below decks in the boiler room, bailing out water that is up to their waists—or wastes.

At this point Kel wakes up and asks how I'm doing. When I tell him about the dream and the meditation that becomes imagery, he asks whether the kidneys are frantic. No, just working really hard. And then he says, "I think you don't need to find your friend Mary at the conference; you know the answer to your own question. You're moving from Surviving to Sustaining." Snuggling up to Kelly in with the heart-to-heart exchange that we learned in the workshop, I know that my tears are truly ones of gratitude, awe, and love.

I am so swept up in the glowing Jedi image that I do not take into account that Mary didn't make it to the Sustainable Living workshop because she ran out of time when my dream ended.

Genetics: The Limitations of a Targeted Approach

During a trip to see Eric, Kylie, and Aidan, Tarceva interacts with something, and for the second time since Aidan was born my eyes are so swollen I can barely see. Is Tarceva worth this? Is it even still helping? The cancer has grown twice already on its watch. Could my own body do a better job preventing the cancer from reoccurring if it was restored to full strength without Tarceva forcing my liver to run marathons and my kidneys to continuously bail water?

That afternoon I receive an unsolicited call from a thoracic oncologist from Memorial Sloan Kettering in New York.

He wants to recruit me for a study exploring why never-smokers get cancer. Because of my previous colon cancer I don't qualify for the trial, but while the oncologist is on the phone, I grab the opportunity to ask him if Memorial Sloane Kettering has had any patients go off of Tarceva. He says he recommends staying on it because after some patients have gone off Tarceva the cancer has progressed quite quickly. But he cautions me that he can't speak to my case specifically.

I go back into meditation to continue to listen to my body. This time my colon is the first one to show up.

Colon woman: I don't trust you.

Me: Nice to meet you, too. Well, I don't trust you, either. I can barely go out without you giving me diarrhea for hours.

Colon woman (upping the ante): You cut me in half!

Me (shouting): Well you gave us cancer, and threatened the whole rest of the body!

Colon woman pouts.

Me (looking to salvage the conversation): But this isn't going to help. Let's hug. (We do, and it's a nice, long hug.)

Colon woman (breaking the hug abruptly): Nuts.

Me (coming slowly out of how good the hug felt and thoroughly bewildered): Nuts?

Colon woman, with a brusque nod of her head: And berries.

Me (laughing at this turn of the conversation): Oh, so now, we're negotiating. OK to the nuts and berries, but we've got to add chocolate.

Colon woman: Done.

Apparently negotiate is a key word, because suddenly we're all in a conference room, me at the head of the table, Colon Woman at the foot. The rest of my organs are lined up on the right and left according to their position in the body. Liver Man won't sit down, however; he's either pacing or leaning against the whiteboard on the right side of the room.

'Kidneys? You OK?' I ask.

'Yes,' they answer, 'but we'd like more water please.'

We're about to continue this meeting in an orderly fashion when in walks the Goddess Immune System supporting Left Lung Woman (LLW since we're in a corporate board room, where acronyms are trendy) by the arm, as LLW moves gingerly to the table. Recognizing that she is frail and vulnerable, all the other organs immediately stop their conversations and start beaming her with energy and light. She responds immediately, transforming into her young self. The organs think it best to do the same for Right Lung Woman (RLW), which they do, and the meditation ends.

Reflecting on this, I decide that my organs believe that protecting and enhancing the left lung is still the priority, and the other organs are okay. So I'll stay on the Tarceva for a while longer.

My dream that night is one of satellite dishes listening to my inner-terrestrials.

⊙ ⊙ ⊙

Ironically, just when I've been considering going off Tarceva, Genentech's PR firm contacts me about the possibility of becoming a media spokesperson for them. It turns out I don't qualify because I am "off-label": Dr. Eaton's decision to prescribe me Tarceva *before* chemotherapy was genius, not protocol. But the PR person does give me the name of another survivor, who has given them permission to do so.

I call her immediately. She did have traditional chemo and radiation before beginning Tarceva, but here's what else she did: she listened to Dr. Weil's tapes, ate organic, visualized, prayed, journalled, drank smoothies, and felt the support of what she calls thousands. What about her family?

"My husband was desperate, and wanted to find anything he could to keep me alive. He researched and taught himself Reiki. He was proud that he felt so much energy in his hands. Now that I've been well so long, he doesn't do it any more and I miss it."

"What do you think was the most important thing for your survival?" I ask.

"I'll let you talk to him," she says, handing over the phone.

"I saved her," says her six-year old son, who was two when she was diagnosed. I believe him.

We're an informal clinical trial of two for the power of Tarceva combined with music, good diet, supportive friends, a husband's loving hands, and a two-year-old in our lives. Scientists like to say that "the plural of anecdote is not data," but to someone dangling on the edge of the bell curve, the plural of anecdote is company.

"I've got to run, I've got band rehearsal." She's a music teacher. But she also has colitis. Perhaps it's genetic, since her sister also has it, but I can't help worrying that it might be a delayed effect of Tarceva. The more I become attuned to the synchrony of the systems in my body, the more I start to worry about the cost of interfering with them. Should I continue with Tarceva? Beth Israel and Memorial Sloan Kettering (MSK) suggest their patients stay on it indefinitely, but on his GRACE website Dr. Jack West from Swedish Hospital says the evidence is scant for this approach. Doctors are apparently continuing Tarceva because they have few other options, not because there's any science to back it up. One doctor from the Cleveland Clinic puts it this way when I post a question on the blog about my concerns:

> I don't believe anyone has published on the long-term side-effects of this treatment so it is impossible to say if there could be long-term consequences. The issue of long-term toxicity is not a problem that anyone ever thought would be an issue in advanced NSCLC patients, but is a good one to have!

Sarri is right, we are still in the Unknown.

⊙ ⊙ ⊙

Perhaps all this discussion wasn't about whether I would leave Tarceva but whether it was leaving me. The spots were not ditzels, they were the result of a new mutation, just like my stem cell meditation had pointed out, and Tarceva is not effective against it. But before I tell you the rest of the story, let's take a moment to consider where we stand in March 2009, nearly three years after I was given three months to live. Leading-edge technology, Tarceva and GammaKnife, combined with the ancient healing protocols of love, joy, touch, and meditation pushed my cancer into retreat for nine months and kept it from significantly advancing for nine more; CyberKnife, a still experimental technology with the power of a linear accelerator, got what it aimed for and gave me nine additional months of progression-free survival; then total immersion in a sea of energy, where organs talk and the world as I knew it shattered to reveal a brilliant, multi-dimensional universe underneath, gave us nine months more.

CHAPTER NINE

Anatomy of a Cellular Conversation

March–April, 2009

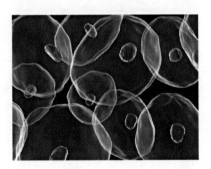

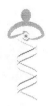 *Kel and I are getting an insider's look at a new airplane still on the drawing boards. We review the blueprints up on the wall. Then we are in Dr. Eaton's room, waiting for him to come in. He enters.*

Dr. Eaton: Your tests are good but…

Me (interrupting): What is it?

He shoots me in the back with what looks like a gun, but the bullet acts more like a dart. Instead of killing me, it propels me into the moonscape of my lungs. Walking over a small hill, I come upon a dark body of water. Suddenly the new high-tech plane whose plans Kel and I had just seen flies in and lands. The nose of the plane extends down and starts sucking out the water.

Sitting on a bench on top of the plane with other observers looking over his shoulder, the pilot operates the nose of the plane remotely, like a steam shovel operator manipulating his bucket.

I wake up the next morning, on March 22, knowing the cancer is back and believing that Dr. Eaton will recommend video-assisted thoracic surgery (VATS)—a procedure in which the surgeon operates from a distance using a robotic arm. Two days later, this is exactly what happens. Dr. Eaton walks into the examining room and says, "Your blood test looks fine." But just as I did in the dream, I can see from his body language that he has more to say. Time slows as I wait for his next sentence: "But your tumor is growing."

There's the shot in the back.

"You're what's known in the profession as an 'interesting case.' Now usually this designation doesn't work to the patient's benefit but in your case, it does. You've gone three years without metastasis. As far as we know, there is no cancer elsewhere. Maybe I'm crazy but I'm going to put your case before the UW Tumor Board with a recommendation for surgery, possibly followed by chemo and radiation."

"With what intent?" I ask. After three years, I am hoping the word palliative will be replaced. I hold my breath.

"Curative," he says. I don't know if he registers how significant this moment is for me. I never thought he would use this word in my presence.

I tell him about my plane dream two nights ago, and my premonition that he would recommend VATS. Is that what he's saying? Or could we accomplish the same thing with another round of targeted radiation like I had with CyberKnife? I'm concerned that the enormity of the surgery might compromise my immune system during the long recovery.

"Yes. I am recommending VATS. We have the leading expert in VATS surgery, Dr. Mike Mulligan, here. He makes it a point of pride to do the least harm. And in the meantime, you can check with Dr. Mehta about CyberKnife."

Kel and I walk out of the office feeling calm. My dream previewed this entire scenario right down to *Mike Mulligan & His Steam Shovel*. Kel immediately makes the adjustment, too. We both look at each other and say, "It's time to re-immerse." As we drive home, Kelly glances over at me frequently for signs of shock. When he finds them he drives past the exit to the ferry and heads north, to the blooming tulip fields where nature dressed in rich purples, reds, and oranges is waiting to share its healing power.

◉ ◉ ◉

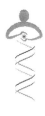

*I am going to perform underwater dancing. I know I have
no training in this form, but I've been asked to do it and
I think I can. I ask Sarri if she agrees, and she nods. I ask
Eric and he answers, 'Sure you can do it, Mumsy, but
how about practicing on dry land first?' So he and I start
waltzing on a patio by the ocean.*

*Kel joins us and then Isaac, Camilla, Thea, Jasper, Kylie,
and Aidan in a long line that extends into the ocean. We
all hold hands, treading water. When a big wave comes
I cry out, 'Hold onto the babies!' and it passes under us
without incident.*

'That wasn't so bad,' we say to each other.

This second dream, the night after the plane dream, sets up the questions I will spend the next few weeks trying to resolve: Should I have the surgery Dr. Eaton recommended? Stick with a western medical intervention but try radiation again instead? Or deepen my internal conversation, increase my level of Qigong practice, and try to dance underwater?

What *was* underwater dancing? I wonder. Was it what we'd been doing for the last nine months, but had lost focus on, or was there a new dance we needed to learn? What seems most fundamental about underwater dancing is that the very thing dancers count on—how gravity applies—is different underwater. What goes up does not necessarily come down, and how you move and push off is not the same. You don't have to go to the cellular level to experience the world in a fundamentally different way; a quick dip in the waters of our own planet is enough.

To: My wonderful support team
From: Diana
Date: March 25, 2009
Subject: It's back. We're back.

Hi wonderful support team,

We found out yesterday that the cancer is growing again on that little spot we all successfully arrested last summer. It appears to be growing slowly so we have at least a month before we'll take any action. There is "opportunity" in this "crisis." My doctor said because I remain strong, fit, and asymptomatic with no metastasis in 3 years, he is going to take my case before the tumor board as a possible candidate for surgery. We'll see my CyberKnife radiologist on Monday, and he has a CyberKnife2 option that we'll discuss. And there's a pill (Tarceva2) that will hopefully start clinical trial in 3 months. So there are options.

But I'd just as soon skip them all and do what we do best. (Apparently having a spot that didn't grow last summer wasn't enough "proof" for the universe, so we have to go through this little exercise again with a demonstrably growing spot.) Are you still up for helping? If you are (you can cite caregiver fatigue and opt out without anyone being the wiser), then please send instructions from your healthy lung cells to mine on how to recognize and neutralize cancer cells.

How, you ask? Just beam light—the instructions will come along with it. I've got a circle of healing energy running 24/7 an inch below my clavicle that is acting as the love port. We've all had so much experience in sending and receiving by now that I know we will succeed. But as Malcolm Gladwell says in his book *Outliers: The Story of Success*, no one—not a musical prodigy, software entrepreneur, or financial wizard—does it alone. And I am very grateful for all you've done to get me through this.

My heart is full with my love for you,
Diana

It has been 35 months, but it still amazes me how much connection and love I can feel in my friends' replies to my email. In most cases we're way past their comfort level (and some choose to make no response as a result, I'm sure). Yet many do reply. Some folks are religious and add me to their prayers. Some are spiritual and invoke help from the universe. But I'm confounded by how many, without a clear philosophy for how this will help, vow to send me healing energy nevertheless.

So this morning, as I reply to each friend, I take a minute to close my eyes, thank them from my heart for the generosity of their spirits, and try to absorb what each is giving me. Because here's the fascinating thing: even in email everyone seems to have an energetic signature that is as unique and legible as their electronic signature. Heartfelt singing. Deep warmth. Restrained worry. Playful and encouraging. Wise and reassuring. Bounding like Tigger. I know that even when the message is brief, my friends are doing what they can to send me something useful. Bypassing conscious thought, their messages are transmitting directly and deeply into my cells; my new source code is being written.

Kel, of course, requires no recruiting. He puts his hands on either side of my lungs and we both feel a powerful current between us, a heat that shines deep into the cancer. We sense in our bodies a ball of light with intelligence around it, working, working, figuring it out.

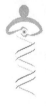

Thea and I are sitting in two wooden children's chairs in an open white space. Thea sits in the right chair with her healthy cells piled to the right of her. I sit in the left chair with my cancerous cells piled to my left. It is story time, but instead of me reading to Thea, she is reading to me from the Book of DNA. Now it is my turn to be the one who asks all the persistent questions of a three-year-old: Why? Why? Why?

Looking across the room I see a woman skeleton in a chair. So death, too, is here.

Coming To a Crossroads

When I first heard about the Seattle Cancer Care Alliance, I was very impressed by the concept of a Tumor Board. The best minds from the member hospitals would gather around a table and work together to find a solution.

"I just got out of the Tumor Board meeting," says Dr. Eaton. "I'm not so sure what I think about it. When you're 1 in a 100, or 1 in a 1,000, there is no science, there's just a bunch of opinions sitting around a table."

"Did those opinions reach any conclusion?" I ask.

"Surgery's worth a try."

Dr. Mulligan was out of town presenting at a VATS surgery conference and missed the Tumor Board meeting. He's less than impressed with its conclusion. "The Tumor Board gives the tough cases to the guy who's out of the room," he says.

"Would I be better off having another round of radiation targeted at this new mass now, and save a surgery option for later?" I ask as I show him a study comparing surgery to stereotactic radiation.

"I'm trying to bite my tongue here," he says. Spare the tongue, I think, your body language is already doing a great job of communicating.

He tells me that any more radiation would absolutely preclude any surgery option later. He's not even sure that the current state of my blood vessels after the CyberKnife dose I've already received will allow surgery. He's afraid that one of my blood vessels might simply disintegrate when his instruments touch it, leaving him unable to suture it back together.

That's it for our conversation. He's paged out of the room.

"That didn't go so well," I explain to Dr. Eaton on the phone. "I think I offended him by mentioning the study."

"Don't worry, I'll talk to him," says Dr. Eaton. "Go see Dr. Mehta and call me back."

⊙ ⊙ ⊙

In contrast, Dr. Mehta is smiling.

"The PET/CT is fantastic. It shows only two spots on the lung, and no other evidence of distant disease. Because of where those spots are, and because there are only two, local therapy—either surgery or radiation—is now an option. Surgery has the advantage of being all done, lobe out and cancer gone. It is the more definitive of the two."

"Is CyberKnife even an option again?" I ask.

"CyberKnife is a brand name. This time we would recommend another stereotactic radiation technology that could be done without implanting the markers that caused you trouble last time. The radiation would take place over a few more sessions. As I say, both surgery and radiation are reasonable options."

"What are the risks of each?" I ask.

"The risk in radiation is underlying lung damage: you could get either pneumonia or a fibrosis reaction in the area. In most cases, the amount of fibrosis is less than what surgery causes, but sometimes the pneumonia can cascade. That risk is small, and we typically treat it with steroids over a relatively short course. This is worst case. With surgery, you can expect pain and a longer recovery."

"Does surgery put my immune system at risk?"

"That's an interesting question. We do know that cancer cells circulate through the bloodstream during surgery. That's been proven. But we don't know whether that makes a difference. It has not been shown that the cancer actually lands anywhere."

"What are the advantages to both approaches?"

"The advantage of radiation is that it's not surgery. The

disadvantage is also that it's not surgery: you don't get the satisfaction (for what it's worth) that the cancer is out and in a bucket. It's a bit challenging to make this decision. In my mind, the reason you go through the pain of surgery is because the cancer ends up in the bucket and you're gold-stamped cured. But in your case we may never get to stamp it, so is it worth it? How uncomfortable are you with the unknown?"

Did he really just ask me that question? "I *live* in the unknown."

Dr. Mehta nods. "So the question is, what is the nature of this disease? Is it that it has metastasized everywhere but Tarceva has kept it under control? If so, we would need another systemic agent like chemotherapy. But if we think the risk of the cancer being in your lung is higher than the risk of it being in the rest of your body, then surgery is an option."

"None of us knows the answer to this question," I reply.

"No, we don't," he agrees. "I think that the risk of it coming back is greater in your lung than anywhere else, but I don't necessarily think the risk is only in this area. The risk is where the cells were the day you were diagnosed, which in your case included your lymph nodes, both lungs, and brain. As a result, the realist would say that any place in your body could be at risk. But if you subscribe to a different theory—that it's all gone but the two points in the one lobe—then surgery is more definitive. If you want to believe that potentially you could be cured, then I believe that, too. The reality is nobody knows."

I ask him about Dr. Mulligan's concern that the blood vessels are too fragile after the high dose of radiation I've received.

"The concern is valid, but the question is do we have anything to back it up? How many surgeons have actually operated on a patient after CyberKnife? It's fundamentally different than low-dose radiation every day for 5–6 weeks. Knowing the CyberKnife centers throughout the country as I do, I am not sure that any surgeon has ever operated on a patient with lungs that have received the high-dose single shot that you've had."

He takes a deep breath. "I look at you. I want to be optimistic and hopeful that this spot is the only place that cancer remains in your body. If that's the case, then removing it makes sense, because then it's gone. The realist in me asks how many stage IV patients have we cured? And if that's the thought process, what's the probability that you're the first?"

Kel interjects: "And she *would* be the first?"

"Unless you've heard of others with similar stories." He looks squarely at Kel and then back to me.

"I want to believe," I answer his unspoken question. "How many people have you seen like me?"

"I only see lung cancer patients. Five of them are three-year survivors, and none are cured five and ten years out. That's not to say that you won't be the first in a tidal wave of people." He leans forward to encourage me. "How is it that you are here with this opportunity? You've already won. You're sitting in that chair right now. You're 1 in 100, 1 in 1000. You've done very well with your decisions. The surgeon is doing surgery that he hasn't performed before; we scare ourselves each time we try new things."

He starts to recap: "You couldn't possibly have a better PET scan. Touch back with Dr. Eaton and listen to what your gut tells you. It makes a lot of sense to consider surgery. There is a reality here that this may not be your last scare. So be it, it beats the alternative of not having survived this long.

"Let me give you one last thought for the surgery team," he says. "Ask them if they are treating you because they believe they are going to cure you. Ask them if they want to be part of the 1 in 1,000 Club."

It would be great to have the opportunity to ask Dr. Mulligan these questions, but after we wait for two hours hungry, needing to pee, and freezing in the examining room without anyone explaining the delay, he's a no-show, and we're left to talk with an intern.

Questions, and More Questions

After meeting with the doctors, I start to draw a decision chart (just like Benjamin Franklin did when he was deciding on a wife): neat columns labeled Surgery, Radiation, Chemo, and Nothing across the top and Risks, Benefits, and Recovery down the side. And that's as far as I get. Because I can't fill in the chart.

Until I was diagnosed I had assumed that any medical evidence I would need would exist and that my medical team would either know it or find it. I hadn't given much thought to whether medical evidence could be waylaid by bias, marketing agendas, or outright fraud. I didn't know enough to evaluate whether the science behind the evidence was well-designed and statistically relevant. And I really hadn't considered what would happen if there wasn't any evidence at all, much less evidence pertinent to my disease and applicable to me.

At this crossroads, there not only isn't any documented path, apparently there isn't even a precedent. This decision simply cannot be reached as a result of linear thinking. We are all dipping into our intuitions: the Tumor Boards' that surgery was "worth a try" and Dr. Mulligan's that he would be able to handle what he hadn't seen before. But Dr. Mehta's fundamental question—*What was the nature of this cancer?*—could not be determined by a chart, a study, or any known cancer diagnostic tool. Is this the moment to trust my intuition again and let my body be the expert? I think *yes*. But will the definitive imagery come to me and will I understand what it's truly trying to tell me?

So far, the answer is *no* and I'm back on Sarri's couch.

"Sarri, what does it mean for me to now be in the 1 in 1,000 Club? Do I just do ten times more of whatever I'm doing? Or does it mean I've got to stretch the limits of what my senses tell me, and shed any preconceptions around what I do?"

I'm catching Sarri up on all the doctor visits and delight her with Dr. Mehta's question of how comfortable am I with the unknown.

"You've already been walking in the unknown. What preconceptions do you think you need to shed now?" she asks.

"I've been working with the two known approaches to cancer: prevent it or eliminate it. Now I'm thinking of a third: transform it. I keep reading articles where scientists describe cancer cells as cunning, resilient, adaptable, and above all, cooperative. But if these cells are so damned adaptable, so capable of learning, why can't they learn to live without destroying me, to limit their unrestrained growth so I won't have to destroy them through surgery, radiation, or chemotherapy? I am willing to live with them if they are willing to live with me."

"What do you think they're like? Can you personify them like you did Anxiety?" she asks.

"Well, some scientists call cancer cells 'immature,' which conjures up an image of the teen-age boys who joined my high school productions halfway through their senior year." Sarri knows some of them. Never having been in a musical before, they didn't really comprehend the need for rehearsing, and they certainly weren't grasping that their failure to learn their parts would have a harmful impact on their self-image and the whole production. This realization typically dawned during tech rehearsal: One night before dress rehearsal, two days before opening night, these boys would look at me with wide, glassy eyes, speechless with terror.

"But something happened during those two days. Somehow a

miracle always occurred. They transformed from high school boys, lonely heroes in their own worlds, into starring members of an ensemble. Unfailingly, after the curtain dropped on opening night, they jumped and whooped in their exhilaration. They even hugged the old lady who directed them. Maybe my cancer cells could go through the same transformation. A hug would be nice, Sarri."

She laughs.

"Seriously, this is all I'm thinking about. Can cancer cells revert to healthy cells? Or is it the healthy cells that need to 'grow up' and take more responsibility for keeping their neighborhoods healthy? How do you do something like turn on a tumor suppressor gene? And are we evolving as a species to be able to have more control over our bodies' inner workings?"

Sarri knows I don't expect her to answer. Gently reeling me in, she asks, "What are your dreams telling you?"

I share what I can remember of my last night's dream and how it ended with two hands around my neck.

"Diana, you're so much stronger than you were last year. You are the captain of your ship, and you are listening. I think your dream means that sadness and fear also want you to listen to them," Sarri suggests. "Are you afraid the surgery might be life-threatening?"

I nod.

"Is Kelly?" she asks compassionately.

"I don't think so. Kelly heard Dr. Mulligan say that he might open me up and not be able to continue the operation if he saw my blood vessels were too fragile. But I heard Dr. Mulligan say he might start operating and not be able to stop the bleeding if a vessel disintegrated at his touch."

Perhaps this is too close to home because I change the subject and start to tell Sarri what happened when Kel and I drove home from the doctor's appointment. On a whim Kel followed two eagles from the highway to the bluffs of nearby Ebey's Landing. When we got there, ten eagles were in view! For an hour we watched their courtship ritual: how they lock talons, somersault, and free-fall, pulling up at the last possible second.

Sarri realizes that while last year I wanted to untie the emotional ropes that bound me into old patterns, now I want to both tie in to my cells and out to universal energies. "Didn't you tell me once that in both the Native American and Qigong traditions, if you come across an unusual event in nature, you can think of it as a guide?" Sarri's right. To the western mind an occurrence in nature is viewed as coincidence, but according to shamanic tradition and the Chinese Yi Jing it could be viewed as correspondence.

"What were you asking those ten eagles?" she says.

"Does the universe want me to live?" I reply. "I took the unusual number of eagles to be a yes. Then, when we started to walk down the beach an eagle hovered just 50 feet away from us for almost a minute. We've never experienced anything like this in our twenty years on Whidbey. The connection seemed so personal that I asked, 'Will you take this cancer from me?' and again I think the answer was yes."

Sarri nods in that non-committal way therapists have perfected.

"Here's another funny eagle story," I continue. "I was talking yesterday morning with friends about 'Who is my teacher? What do I need to learn, and who do I need to I learn it from right now? Is there some spiritual practice that could provide an answer?' And then yesterday afternoon as Kel and I walked the bluffs, yet another eagle came up the cliff directly behind me and- flew to the tree just ahead."

Sarri smiles despite herself.

"So Kel and I stop. 'Okay, eagle, if you're volunteering to be my teacher, I'll wait for your guidance.' I open up my palms to receive this communication and stand there. And stand there. And stand there. Kel lies down in the grass to wait with me. Do you know how long eagles can perch in a tree? For freaking ever! After 45 minutes I got antsy and decided to try to touch the tree, at which point it flew away."

"What lesson did you learn?" asks Sarri, laughing at my dramatic reenactment of the scene.

"Be patient."

"Diana, your questions aren't just about whether or not to have surgery—they are life's big questions, and you can't get answers until you can be more precise. Why don't you make a list?"

And so I do. In a stream of consciousness I type out 108 points to consider.

Waiting For My Body's Orders

Thea, in her first foray as a flower girl, is thoughtfully dropping one rose petal at a time onto the path that her Aunt Sarah will soon walk down. Thea's three-year old cousin, Emmett, the ring-bearer, thinks that looks like fun. He grabs the basket from Thea and starts throwing petals; she grabs back, and they both start throwing fistfuls until Emmett turns the basket over, dumps all the petals, runs away from the congregation, and rolls in the grass.

"What do I do now, Dad?" Thea asks, still at the end of the aisle.

"Pretend you're still throwing petals and afterwards come sit up in front next to me," Isaac replies.

Weddings don't always go as planned, just like life. Laughter trumps planning, but Thea's question is still relevant to me. What do I do now? I've been patiently waiting for days for the definitive communication, dream, or meditation to guide me. Each morning brings multiple dreams that I scribble on the margins of the Super

Sudoku book by my bed. Cutting through a hedge. Trying to find a path. Choosing between fancier and more comfortable shoes. Cold feet. The only meaning I can take from these dream fragments is that the answer I seek still eludes me.

My meditations are clearer but no less indecisive, although my attitude toward the cancer is transforming.

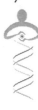

The Goddess holds me, one hand on my head and one on my abdomen. We are in a circle with a teenage boy on our left and an adult woman on our right. He is the cancer. She is the upper lobe of my lung. I recognize her from yesterday's meditation.

I realize it's not appropriate for me to judge the boy and the woman. Instead we are waiting to know them, to see who they are. The Goddess and I show them compassion by holding them as we sit nested with one another facing the view. We break apart to stand overlooking the canyon on the edge of the glen, the boy and the woman on either side of the Goddess and me. 'Are they part of this future?' the Goddess and I wonder.

When I look at the teenage boy, I realize that he isn't aggressive, malicious, or egotistical. He is a boy, like my nephews and the teenage boys I've shepherded through musicals. I think I can teach him, but whether he wants to stay in the glen is an open question.

Maybe returning to music is the way to an answer. Kel and I go to the Seattle Symphony to see Vadim Repin, a world-class violin soloist. As the sound cascades over me, it strikes me how many notes there are in this virtuosic performance of the Brahms Violin concerto in D, which reminds me of the unimaginable number of cells in my body: 100 trillion cells in the body, 1 trillion in the brain alone.[87]

So I start doing some math in my head. How many people are there in the world right now? Nearly 7 billion. Imagine town squares the world over filled with people dancing the same choreography, like a spontaneous event on YouTube. Even if the feat of getting all humans to collaborate were possible, we only comprise 7 billion entities. How many individual mammals are there? How many species do you have to include in the animal kingdom—birds, reptiles, fishes?—before you reach 100 trillion individuals? Would they all work together if their survival depended on it? How would they communicate with each other, and I with them?

And yet Mr. Repin and every other musician in front of me are living proof that trillions of cells *can* collaborate in astonishing harmony to create healthy people, world-class musicians, and Olympic athletes. Will they let me join the conversation? I feel my cells are trying to do just that, yelling like the Whos in Dr. Seuss' Whoville, trying to reach me with the news that they *will* cooperate for the good of the whole, and that my role is to be their voice: to serve them rather than them serve me. Maybe the goddess image wasn't so far off. Perhaps we are all god-like figures responsible for far more life than we can see with our naked eyes.

I'm in tears by the time the concert is over. I am the voice of my 100 trillion cells and if I don't speak for them, who will? But what are they asking of me?

Perhaps to fundamentally change who I think I am. What if this sense of "I" is not the basic unit? What if what I perceive as "I" is simply a mouthpiece for my cells, who need an advocate to act on their behalf while they toil in a watery environment sensing, responding, and reacting according to very different rules of perception, engagement, and motion than the world I experience?

If I am going to dance underwater, I'm going to have to be a good dance partner. My cells will lead, and I will follow.

⊙ ⊙ ⊙

Kel and I set out on a meandering meditation to fill my cells with the healing power of euphoria. It's easy to believe this is possible when the spring sun is first reaching Seattle, and with a mighty exhalation we expel winter and worry from our collective lungs and psyches. I'm waiting for the inhalation after that, which smells so sweet that the lungs slow in appreciation.

We return to Total Immersion. Our hands clasped together, Kel and I feel the love pulsing and energy building between us as we walk downhill to the Bainbridge ferry. We savor the brashness of the yellow daffodils, the elegant invitation to spring extended by the pink magnolias. We drink in the beauty of the white-capped Puget Sound and the snow-capped Olympic mountains in the distance, trying to bring awe all the way in to the cellular level.

We follow intuition. An abrupt and arbitrary right turn halfway down the Harbor Steps takes us into a yoga studio we've never even noticed before. Within minutes we are in a private session with its spiritual leader. Instead of climbing the rugged Himalayas to find the yogi on the mountaintop, we've just strolled down an urban hill, but perhaps he's just the teacher I need at this moment. His energy is certainly serene, gentle, and sweet. It feels good to be here with him, but Kelly and I aren't sure whether to giggle or goggle.

Kel and I agree to come back for what the teacher calls a healing session. We're not expecting a cure, but all of our intention goes to hoping this will make a difference. When we return and my healing session begins, my intuitively accessed instructor sits cross-legged beside me as I lie stretched out on a mat in a dimly lit room. He places his hand on my abdomen and starts to move my muscles in a slow, gentle, soothing motion. His hand accelerates in a tight circle, the pressure light on my skin. What's this about? The teacher's body starts swaying in a wide circle, his hands on my belly increasing their pressure and their speed. When is this going to stop? His body arches over me, putting more weight on my abdomen. I hope this is almost over. Faster still, harder. Yow, make this stop! But it doesn't. Okay, I give up, I surrender. I go somewhere else, deep into the healing glen where my goddess and I stand looking at the view of my future.

The answer I've been waiting for pops out in my mind and at almost exactly the same moment the teacher stops his motion.

"Are you satisfied with your decision?" he asks.

Am I satisfied with my decision? That's an interesting question, but the wrong one. It doesn't matter whether I'm satisfied. What matters is whether or not I believe that this is what my body ordered. And of that I have no doubt. The images are too clear and too compelling. I have trusted them before and I know that this is the moment to trust them again.

To: My wonderful support team
From: Diana
Date: April 15, 2009
Subject: Re: Going for it

Hi wonderful support team,

Well, we have decided to go "for the cure," for the "hail Mary pass," for surgery. This is an opportunity that with your help I have "earned" by virtue of no metastasis for three years and being in great shape. Kel and I met with the surgeon, radiologist, and oncologist, and all three recommended surgery, even though it falls outside everyone's experience and no one can say with certainty that it will work as a cure. All of them agreed that ultimately I would have to consult my body to make the decision, and that it had served me well so far.

After a lot of convoluted dreams, and meetings with docs, healers, therapist, and family, my meditation showed me and my inner healer looking at my future (a very expansive view, by the way). All of a sudden my chest opened up, the upper lobe of my lung popped out and landed on the ground, and the healer reached into my open chest wound to stop the bleeding and start the healing. In case I missed that message, the scene shifted: everyone in the family reached into a bowl to pull out a slip of paper and every one said "surgery." I guess if you don't listen to poetic imagery, you just get the message straight.

I asked whether anyone at the UW wants my tumors and lung to study. Apparently a non-smoker that has responded to Tarceva—and responded as well as I have—is the "Holy Grail," as the woman who asked me to sign the consent form said, so I will be patient #1 in their tissue bank. I'm very excited by the thought that this journey of ours could help others in the future.

Much love and appreciation,
Diana

In 1959, my grandmother died of lung cancer. According to family lore, she was never told she had it. Her cancer was too advanced, and there was no known treatment: better not to upset her. A revolution in the doctor-patient relationship has taken place between her diagnosis and mine. My cancer also was too advanced, and there was still no known cure, but not only was I being told, I would be the one to make the decisions.

I have thought often about why this is a step forward. I don't have the training that my doctors do, and by spelling out the prognosis so clearly, we add to my stress levels and thereby lose a critical advantage from the placebo effect. Perhaps fear of malpractice drove doctors to change this relationship, but what do I, the patient, bring to the table that makes it an advantage for me?

When Drs. Eaton and Rockhill laid out my first treatment options, I didn't have the background to do anything but rely on their judgment. My contribution to the cause was merely having chosen them. I quickly realized this ability to choose implied that I, not my doctors, was the team leader. I would be the one to recruit who was on the team and how big it was. I started with myself, Kel, my family, and my friends, and over time I added skilled practitioners from both the medical and integrated healing communities.

Another good reason to include me in the decision-making was that I alone knew how much I could and would contribute to healing by taking care of my body, emotions, and spirit, and what I was willing to endure physically. In the age of the Internet, I was even able to research and suggest a treatment, CyberKnife, that had been outside the box until my doctors were willing to pull it in. But now that I realize I am the voice of my cells, I truly know why my input is so valuable. I am the only one who can truly speak for their point of view. My decision-making process might not be straightforward, but it has gotten the job done, at least so far.

Sanctuary

Even after a dozen or more visits, we're still not completely convinced this place actually exists in any real sense. Envisioned by a guy with a 500-year plan, the Earth Sanctuary is 70-some acres of pure meditation, a spiritual sampler of disparate traditions that includes a Neolithic-style dolmen, a couple of stone circles, Native American prayer sites, Tibetan prayer wheels and strings of prayer flags, a mile or so of trails that wind through the woods and around the fen bog, and a small, three-circuit left-handed classic labyrinth made of flagstone path bordered with native plants. It's just what we are looking for.

No one else is here. We spend the morning in self-imposed silence, surrounded by the non-verbal speech of resident wildlife. We observe each tradition as we come to it. Ducks land on the pond as we do our Qigong on the bank. We smudge ourselves with sage. The towering Stonehenge-like circle of twelve columns of Columbia River Basalt looks like the circle of organ systems in my first meditation, so I know just what to do here. I go into the center of the circle and feel the light. After this we walk the labyrinth: emptiness on the way in, gratitude on the way out.

Kel gives me a Reiki/Jin Shin treatment on a bench at the end of a very short peninsula midway along the fen. This too is an unreal place, untethered to time or place. It feels to us like we haven't stumbled upon it so much as we've somehow summoned it. And if that's the case, we can get back here if we need to. Without the car.

"Kel, if the pain gets too much during surgery...." I pause.

"I'll meet you here," he says.

To: Small group of South Whidbey friends
From: Diana
Date: May 2, 2009
Subject: A last-minute dress rehearsal

With just a few days to go before my surgery, we would like to invite you to help us prepare for it and my recovery by coming to a Dress Rehearsal tomorrow at 4:00 at our house (sorry for the late notice, we're living pretty much day-to-day). Because I'm such a visual person, we're going to prepare by walking through the surgery.

Then we'll party to celebrate Cinco de Mayo with chicken/bean chili and beer. Does this sound fun?

If you can come, bring nothing but a healthy body and willing spirit. I'm afraid I can't take the risk of getting sick with so few days to go. If you can't join us on such short notice, no worries, I know you are always with me.

Love,
Diana

If I can't prepare for the surgery by connecting with Dr. Mulligan, I'll just have to find another way. I've been visualizing the entire operation for days now, but it hasn't been enough to assuage my misgivings. Yesterday I sat up in bed and typed out the entire sequence as a play for a cast of thirty. Olympic skiers arc and twist their bodies in place with their eyes closed as they visualize the downhill ski course before they get in the starting gate. It's called mental practice and if it helps skiers, dart throwers, pianists, and dancers improve their performance, maybe it will help my body through surgery. I'm also hoping that if I can "see" the operation outside my head, it will finally put to rest the anxiety that remains inside.

So far, now that everyone's gathered on our deck, it seems that I've only succeeded in transferring that anxiety to my friends, as they wonder what oddball experience I'm about to put them through. Kel starts things off. "It is Cinco de Mayo and we are celebrating Mexico's example of defeating an invading army. We are here today surrounded by the power of your love, and we certainly don't plan on following Mexico's example of losing every battle that follows this one."

Everyone is quiet, expectant, doubtful, but willing. I am the one who is nervous and choked up. I have to ask Sarri to sit on the step in front of me so I can rest my hand on her head to ground me when I speak. Sarri has her own words to contribute. "These two stones I'm holding symbolize fear and sadness. If unexamined, they are heavy. But if we take the lessons, truth, and guidance away from the sadness and the fear then we can release these heavy stones. That is what we do. That is our work." After we pass the stones around the circle—some people clearly upset as they do—Kel and I drop the stones over the edge of the balcony.

I ask everyone to play a role in this drama we're creating: to be stand-ins for the cells of all the different organs and systems that will be impacted by the surgery. My friends raise their hands to accept cardboard signs with their roles hastily scrawled on them. The most uncomfortable and reluctant among them ask for an easy role.

"You can all be the esophagus, all you've got to do is open wide. "

"We're good at that," they laugh.

Steve and Debora, medical professionals, take up more challenging posts. "We've got the pleura because we're the only ones who know what it is."

"That's great, because it will be the trickiest area for the surgeon to negotiate."

"Then I'll join that team, too," says Doug, a lawyer.

We move into the house, the archetype for the self. I jump onto the dining room table. Kelly, in his role as Dr. Mulligan, has a straw (stand-in for a tube), a flashlight (stand-in for the video) and a sword (stand-in for the scalpel). We start with the bronchoscopy, a procedure to ensure there is no cancer that the CT couldn't see lurking inside the bronchioles of the lung. Kelly's pantomime of searching the bronchioles includes shining a flashlight down the front of my shirt and following it with his hands. Linda, our office manager, covers her mouth, but not quickly enough to cover her guffaw, and the tension in the room dissolves. Now the party can begin.

We walk through the mediastinoscopy, where Dr. Mulligan will remove my lymph nodes and send them to the pathology lab to be sure there's no cancer there. Andrew, our honorary son, plays the part of the lab technician delivering good news to the operating room by running up to our loft and back, skidding across our wood floor like Kramer in *Seinfeld*.

Me to the Skin sentinels: You may be wrinkly but you have done a wonderful job expelling toxins from my body, protecting me from harm, and opening the right channels so I can feel the energy of the universe and the touch of those I love.

Me to the Lymph node sentinels: You are power machines. You fought cancer within yourselves and then worked to free the rest of the body and lung.

Kelly as Dr. Mulligan and the surgical team: Are you prepared for this procedure?

The Sentinels and me: Yes, we are.

Dr. Mulligan: Will you please open the best path for me?

The Sentinels and me: Yes, we will.

Dana, my friend and a public health nurse, standing in for the recovery team: Can you bring in and energize the healing forces within you and without you to make a full recovery?

The Sentinels and me: Yes, we can.

We all move into the living room, each team taking up their stations as bones, pleura, heart, lungs, immune system, liver, bladder, kidneys, and intestines, as Kel, Dana, and I move among them.

Are you prepared? Yes, we are.

Will you open a path for Dr. Mulligan? Yes, we will.

Can you bring all the resources you need for your recovery? Yes, we can.

After the mock operation is over, we work together on the recovery, and then face the future by looking at the mountains and water out our picture window, shoulder-to-shoulder yet alone, uncertain yet accepting whatever will come to pass. It turns out this is not just about me. We all seem to experience the fragility of the future, yet right now we are content to simply be together in the moment.

Then the party begins. Randy and Gordy sing casually by the hearth while everyone else eats or sprawls in the living room. While I no longer feel the nervousness we all started out with, neither do I feel the giddiness and exuberance of the Love-In three years earlier. The conversation today is thoughtful, about new directions and possibilities, about how grateful we are for the support of our community, and about how, although no one has ever actually thanked their liver before, this is as good a time as any to start.

After everyone leaves I sit on the couch a long time trying to process all the swirling, restless emotions of the evening. I walk into the kitchen to brew a cup of tea, and out of the corner of my eye catch a glimpse of golden light shining on the water. The moon must be setting, I think as I turn my head to look, but there's nothing there. It isn't a reflection of the moon; it is a reflection of my heart. My friends have just built a yellow brick road to my future. Dr. Mulligan, now it's your turn.

A Door Opens

The University of Washington Surgery Pavilion looks like an airport without the giant arrivals and departures boards. Too bad. It would be helpful to know how many flights and delays are still ahead of me. Kel, Camilla, Isaac, and I have already waited for an hour and a half in kindergarten-size chairs, the only ones available. In the rest room a young woman awaiting surgery splashes cold water on her face, clearly in panic. "You're going to do well," I tell her. I know how important it is to carry that belief with you into surgery.

When I'm called the nurse tells us that the family will not be able to accompany me into the pre-surgical area, as they always have in the past. I hug them good-bye at the beginning of a hallway that seems endless. Each step requires the courage to not run back to my family; time suspends. Inwardly I summon those who love me to help, and I glide the rest of the way on their magic carpet. I manage to find words to ask the nurse how many surgeries Dr. Mulligan performs in a day. It can be as many as 16 or 17. No wonder I haven't been able to see him.

The pre-surgery room is outfitted like an ER, many beds separated only by sliding curtains. It runs like a MASH unit. The minute I have my gown on I am swarmed by four different people all preparing me—quickly—for surgery. They are late, they are in a hurry, they don't want to keep Dr. Mulligan waiting. And I have screwed the pooch. As a pre-surgery precaution I have been taking an antibiotic that isn't listed on the nurse's paperwork. I have my iPod with me (although it, too, is against protocol) and I know I need it now.

I put Brahms in one ear while the nurses and residents ask me questions through the other. The anesthesiologist comes in to give me an epidural block in my lung cavity. The first attempt doesn't work. "Can you feel that?" he asks as he pokes me with a needle. That? How about now? He tries again and again. Finally he asks me to sit up, swing my legs to the side of the bed and lean over onto the rolling side table with my head on my arms while he continues to poke and prod from the back. Kelly, I'm going to the Earth Sanctuary right now. I'll see you there. I do my best to retreat into our alternate universe and let all of this chaos run its course without me.

A tap on my shoulder. There's a face peering up at me from under the table. The senior surgical resident who was with Dr. Mulligan at our first and only meeting is bent over at the waist, his hands on his knees, trying to tilt his head under mine.

"Are you the one with the dream?"

"Yes."

"Why did you decide to do the surgery?"

"Because I had another visualization where my lung popped out." He's doubtful, but also intrigued.

"Did Dr. Mehta say he wouldn't do the radiation?"

"No, he said he would, but he told me surgery was worth the risk if I believed it could cure me. My imagery said it would."

"OK, see you in there."

I've gotten through to Dr. Mulligan.

CHAPTER TEN
Practical Spirituality

May, 2009–April, 2010

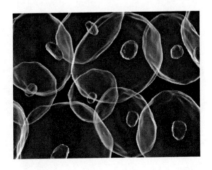

From: Kelly
Date: May 5, 2009
Subject: Cancer-free!

Hello wondrous support team! Nice going on all the prayers, visualizations, meditations, light beaming, Jim Beaming, whatever. It worked fabulously! For the first time in 3+ years, Diana is cancer-free!

The bronchoscopy and mediastinoscopy revealed no surprises, so Dr. Mulligan proceeded with the thoracotomy to remove the upper lobe of Diana's left lung. He said there was considerable scarring from the Tarceva and CyberKnife treatments, which made the surgery extremely difficult and tiring. He admitted that most surgeons wouldn't have attempted the procedure, and those that did probably would've quit halfway through. So we lucked out with the right surgeon and thanked him profusely for persevering. He said essentially that he wanted to push the limits of his profession, for which we are entirely grateful, and even now we in the waiting room are still standing and applauding his chutzpah.

So here's an image for you: lots of critical structures, like blood vessels and airways, all very thin-walled, were wrapped in scar tissue. Dr. Mulligan described this as being like tightly rolled baloney firmly embedded in rawhide—and he had to remove the rawhide without nicking the baloney. It's a difficult image to get your mind around, particularly if you're a vegetarian.

Here's what to visualize for the next few days to weeks, since pain will most likely be Diana's biggest issue. The body has pain gates that open and shut to control the messages to the brain. In her case the brain doesn't need that information because it'll be so obvious why she's in pain, so the constant nagging will just get in the way of healing. So imagine the gates as faucets and dimmer switches. The faucets control the chemical messages; the dimmer switches control the electrical messages. Whenever you think about it—especially tonight and for the next few days—mentally turn off 7 faucets and turn down 7 dimmer switches. That should do it. Many, many thanks, gang!

From: Kelly
Date: May 8, 2009
Subject: A Quick Diana Update

HUGE progress today, after a pretty iffy stretch yesterday. Diana was able to get up and walk after having her blood pressure plummet each time she tried yesterday. There are trade-offs with the drugs so the pain management team is still trying to find the right balance between "No Pain No Gain" and "No Pain Actually Sounds Pretty Good." I grossly underestimated the 7 faucets, though, so for the next day or so just concentrate on a single turnstile that controls the water going over one of the spillways at, say, Hoover Dam. Shut that off instead. The dimmer switches are still good, though.

Love you all. Stay tuned. Goodnight.

From: Kelly
Date: May 11, 2009
Subject: A Very Quick Update on Diana

In the immortal words of Joni Mitchell in the drug-induced haze of the '60s, Diana is now "unfettered and alive"—and still in a bit of a drug-induced haze of her own. They just disconnected the last of the chest tubes and IV so she is now free floating, and at the mercy of oral medication—Dilaudid and Tylenol, not to be confused with Laudanum and Absinthe, which might be equally effective, but scarier.

Thanks for the good work on the turnstiles. It worked so well she had trouble peeing after coming off the catheter. You guys are powerful.

Many, many thanks! Stay tuned.

From: Kelly
Date: May 16, 2009
Subject: Finding our Way Home

What a beautiful day. Blue sky, gorgeous mountains, boats little and big on the water, birds chirping, neighbor's weed whacker whacking... hard to believe how long that thing can go on a little tank of gas.

The final pathology report on the tumor and lymph nodes is good: the lymph nodes and margins are clear, so unless there's something microscopically lurking somewhere (which is always a possibility with metastatic cancer like this), Diana's cancer-free!

We made it back home yesterday afternoon after a bit of a delay picking up more meds and only a one-boat wait to get on the island. Not bad, but still took its toll on Diana. But most of what she describes happening now I see as well, so that's progress. We both see the wild bunnies all over the lawn, only she reports they're wearing tutus.

Our days now are mostly short walks, naps, med schedules, and healing treatments—nothing any more pressing than that. And changing dressings. You wouldn't believe the post-surgical landscape—like some bizarre reverse treasure map of how to get back from somewhere you wish you weren't. I'd attach a photo, but we're thinking of saving it for the Christmas card.

Thanks again for all your help. Love you all.

Travels in the Cuddle Shuttle

Instead of flying to my mother's 80th birthday, we are driving across country in the Cuddle Shuttle, a 2006 Prius we've turned into a micro-RV by folding down the seats and putting a queen-size foam mattress in the back. The mattress is there because I can still only sit up for a couple of hours at a time after the lobectomy. When we stop, the Japanese print window shades and comforter cover we've made lend the illusion of a private Zen garden, when we might in fact be surrounded by tractor-trailer rigs at some rest area on the Interstate.

America is apparently celebrating with us: *America's Recovery and Reinvestment Act* billboards line the roads, pre-announcing the traffic delays for road construction that lie ahead. I'm still under construction too, the trillions of cells in my body collaborating to bring me the healing materials they need to repair a surgery that was never supposed to be within my grasp. They aren't wordless passengers dozing off in the back; they let me know when we need more pain meds with the persistence of a five-year-old yelling are we there yet? Are we there yet? ARE WE THERE YET?

But it's a road trip and we have always loved road trips. We may be celebrating our 35th wedding anniversary, but at heart we are still 21 and heading out to Utah for the first time to celebrate our engagement.

"How many states will we be going through on our way to Connecticut?" Kel asks.

"Seventeen," I answer, after dutifully counting them on the Rand McNally Guide I've started to highlight.

"It's our 35th wedding anniversary, so let's make it 35," he offers, and I'm thrilled to accept. A few more miles roll by in the emptiness of eastern Washington.

Kel starts, "We might as well make it all 50."

I finish his thought, "In how long?"

"Over the course of a year."

"What counts for being in a state?"

"Well, I've been thinking… You know how since we were first married we've always kissed when we cross a state line?" he asks, eyes twinkling.

I start to smile.

"So what do you think a kiss in 1974 would be worth today, adjusted for 35 years of inflation?"

As much as I'm on board with Kel's idea of kiss inflation, I had my doubts about its practicality. I grew up in New England. You can drive through all six states in a single day. That presents a challenge we probably couldn't have met even in our 20s. Yet in our 50s, we decide to try.

Now why would we do this? Because it was the honeymoon

of our new life. Because sex and survival have always gone together. Because it feels good. Because it boosts the immune system.[88] Because it's an antidote to pain. Because it soothes and smooths life and love. Because afterward you snuggle in close to your honey and never want to be anywhere else—unless it's the next state.

But it's not only the "why?" but the "how?" that interests—maybe even confounds—most of our friends. Their questions are less about overcoming the limited space in the Prius and more about how we overcame the assumptions that often limit the role of sex after a certain age. All we can say is that a good sense of humor and letting go of the outcome helps. And a car outfitted like a Geisha parlor doesn't hurt either.

◉◉◉

The current delay finds us at the two-mile-high Beartooth Pass heading into Yellowstone, the most spectacular stretch of highway we've yet seen. We're the first car in line waiting for the pilot car to escort the oncoming traffic through the one-lane mountain pass. "I'm about to wave you through, but you have time to get out of your car and see the view I see everyday," says the flagger. The view is grander than we can articulate.

What is this parallel universe that we have entered? Lose a lobe and all my dreams come true? In this universe my husband wants to travel with me like this for a year. In this universe I can breathe at 9000 feet, hike up a 600-foot elevation gain with lightness and speed, and continually shifting beauty reveals itself in an endless panorama. In this universe I don't have to wish for anything, because what I get is so much more than I would have presumed to ask for.

I like it here, and I'm grateful for the absence of some things that don't seem to have crossed over. Resentments, grievances, duty, and stress all seem to be no-shows. Kel suggests that maybe the lobe was where all my nightmares were stored. We linger, letting all the other cars pass us. We are alone in what our senses tell us is the top of the world. And just when I am already amazed by these gifts, along comes a trail just off the road to three alpine lakes with no sign of anyone else. At the last one I just start taking off my clothes before I even get to it, knowing that Kel will be close behind me. I am filled with joy and love. I recognize that this is my natural state, and that if I ever feel differently all I have to do is listen to my inner navigation system to find home.

This universe is not without its trials, however. Dryness is taking over every crease. My intestines remind me that I am not in charge and have much to learn. Pain calls out for my attention if left unattended for more than six hours. But it means I still live in this body I love. This is not a dream under anesthesia.

We know that there are other parallel universes linked to ours. Our friends email us to ask where we are, and if they can come explore with us. Eric and Kylie send us daily pictures of a laughing Aidan so we don't forget them. Camilla and Isaac call, setting a homing beacon to Seattle. Thea tells me, "Nin, when I tell you 'I love you' I just want to say it again and again." I feel the same way, and Kel and I feel that same way about each other. As our tires roll steadily over variable road surfaces, we seal this moment in our hearts and reinforce it in our brains. This universe is real.

After six trips and 364 days, our return flight from Hawaii touches down in Seattle on the 364th day. Final tally: a grand total of 50 states accompanied by a greater appreciation of the mutability of distance, the relativity of time, the infinite wonder of both wide open spaces and what lies between, and the inestimable value of a good cuddle, anytime, anywhere.

Interrupting the Messenger of Pain

Sing along with Carly and me:

> *I haven't got time for the pain.*
> *I haven't got room for the pain.*
> *I haven't the need for the pain.*[89]

Since surgery Kel's iPhone calendar is filled not with the hour-by-hour appointments of a busy, crazed life but with reminders every four to six hours of my dazed life. Current thinking in pain management is to never let pain gain a foothold, never allow it to breach medicine's chemical defenses and create a permanent tunnel into the stronghold of the brain. So Kel's calendar serves as a record of strategic and tactical skirmishes: the post-surgical counter-offensives of epidurals and Dilaudid; the hasty retreat from OxyContin; an abortive attempt to alternate Vicodin and Ibuprofen, followed by full capitulation to Vicodin; the recruitment of long-lasting Aleve and a Lidocaine patch as my body habituates to the meds and requires more help to fight the pain. By late July, a sample day looks like this:

Sunday	July 26, 2009
● Patch off	6:30 PM, Jul 25 to 6:30 PM, Jul 26
● Vicodin 2	2 AM to 6 AM
● Aleve	7 AM to 11 AM
● Patch on	7:15 AM to 7:15 PM
● Vicodin 2	11:30 AM to 3:30 PM
● Vicodin 2	3:30 PM to 7:30 PM
● Patch off	7:15 PM to 7:15 AM
● Aleve	6:40 PM to 10:40 PM
● Vicodin 2	7:35 PM to 11:40 PM

By late August in the Cuddle Shuttle, the calendar shows troop withdrawal and the reinstatement of some R&R:

Thursday	August 27, 2009
● Vicodin 2	7:20 AM to 11:20 AM
● Vicodin 1.5	7:20 AM to 11:20 AM
● Hike Yellowstone Falls	11 AM to 1 PM
● Vicodin 1.5	11:20 PM to 3:20 PM
● Walk Geyser Trail	3 PM to 4 PM
● Vicodin 1.5	5:15 PM to 9:15 PM

In September we decide to start lessening pain's control of my life by taking away its place on the calendar. This fills instead with the good stuff of life—birthdays, weddings, and Great Adventure days with Thea and Jasper, as I move toward painkiller-on-demand rather than on schedule. But pain's absence from the calendar does not mean its absence from my body, and I don't like how it keeps trying to set up its own recurring appointments. In the middle of the night I log onto the Internet searching for some kind of timeline this pain might be following.

"Chronic post-lobectomy syndrome, post-operative pain that lasts for years or a lifetime," is not a reassuring first search result, nor is "60–70% of patients experience it" a comforting first click. The next day, drumming my heels against the exam table yet again, I ask Dr. Eaton if he has a plan for getting me off the pain meds. "Many of my patients never get off of them," he answers gently.

"Well, that's not going to be me."

I believe pain—like anxiety—is a messenger. Since a message about touching a hot fire has to get to the brain immediately, pain is fast, but it is certainly not nuanced. It hogs the conversation and has problems with volume control. But pleasure can force a break in the monologue. Joy in any form (laughter, a grandchild's hug, Kel's touch) can trump pain, but not without complete concentration.

That's hard to maintain, so I was happy for pain meds while my body was under repair. Pain kept reminding me that fines are doubled in a construction zone. Gliding along in the Cuddle Shuttle, I was happy to have Vicodin along for the ride. But as a general rule, I don't like pain meds. I don't feel as good with them as I do without them. Over the decades I've adopted various strategies for dealing with pain, starting with Bradley childbirth classes before Camilla was born. I have deflected pain by breathing through it, and have broken its hold by moving it around my body. I have cancelled out its signal using the sound waves of music. I have distracted it by focusing my attention elsewhere. Jin Shin, acupuncture, and meditation diminished it, as did certain foods. Most importantly, I've learned that my pain and I are not one and the same. My pain does not define me.

I'm inspired by a study I found. Researchers at Stanford placed people with 10 years or more of chronic pain into an fMRI machine where they could see in real-time the blood flow to the specific part of the brain that experiences pain. By simply looking at a picture of a pain-free brain, they could then voluntarily control the blood flow and most importantly, change their perception of pain in the process. "These effects were powerful enough to impact severe, chronic clinical pain" the researchers observed; maybe they would be powerful enough for me, especially when I learn that the patients in the study were able to control their pain without the fMRI machine feedback through the same kind of "mental interventions" that I had been practicing.[90]

But this time I'm not out to be heroic, or to trick, divert, or otherwise displace the legitimate pain of my body's recovery from surgery. I simply believe that needing pain meds has become an old message. It's time for a safe and orderly withdrawal. I want to work on the source of the pain without masking it with meds, and I discover that physical therapy can help.

During my first session the physical therapist examines my scar—looks great for a 12-inch sword slash—and then touches it. Ouch. Ouch. Ouch. Ouch! Before she can start work, the scar needs to be desensitized to pain. She suggests we start slowly by rubbing something soft on it, a Kleenex, a feather, even Kel's fingers. And then she insists I start wearing a bra again.

Sue, a different physical therapist, takes over in the next session. To hell with desensitization, she just starts kneading the scar tissue. Good time to practice labor breathing. But here's the miracle: when she's done I feel better—and not only because she stopped. Sue taught me that I was once again going to have to dismantle the ties that bind, this time from the scar tissue that surgery has left in its wake.

For up to a year following surgery the body continues to lay down scar tissue. It's a powerful bandage for wounds, but it is doesn't have the resiliency of healthy tissue, so if I move and stretch the healthy tissue will stretch with me, and the scar tissue will reach its limit first. The pain I now experience is literally the point of attachment between scar tissue and healthy tissue. The way to stop this pain is to break down the scar tissue (once the wound has healed) through stretching or deep massage. A trained professional knows the preferred direction of the muscle fiber, but if I can reach it, I can do it myself anytime pain flairs up. Even a tennis ball can help.

For the area inside my lung cavity where no hands can reach, I break the scar tissue down through deep breathing. The easiest way to fill my lungs fully is to walk—preferably uphill. Scar tissue can lead to a loss of flexibility, strength, and power.[91] Breaking it down restores all three functions—physically and psychologically.

I continue physical therapy at Seattle Cancer Care for as long as insurance allows. Jill, my friend and masseuse, continues (forever, hopefully) where Sue leaves off. I also have a trusty little massage ball to rub into the nooks and crannies of my ribs if pain returns at an unfortunate time. And I have Kelly to lay his warm hand over the scar and regulate the energy so the primary message coming from my body is one of love, not pain.[92]

I am off the narcotics within two weeks.

☉☉☉

According to Buddhist philosophy suffering is caused by attachment. Detaching, one idea at a time, one emotion after another, is the Buddhist prescription for relieving emotional pain. Sarri and I used the metaphor of untying one rope after another that attached me to ways of being and relating that were unhealthy. Before he could remove my lung, Dr. Mulligan made that metaphor manifest by tediously removing, strand by strand, fiber by fiber, the scar tissue left from Tarceva's conquering march across my lung and the flash and blast of CyberKnife.

Now I can add the ideas of sports medicine to my healing arsenal. Increase range of motion. Stretch and strengthen. Develop balance and awareness. For any pain I might be feeling, I can stretch my point of view, break down my old assumptions—or simply take a deep breath.

☉☉☉

By now, you'd think I would have learned to read a web site with a grain of salt.

> Even after you heal, you might have some limits on how much physical activity you can do. You probably won't be able to do as much as you could before.[93]

Dr. Eaton agrees that this is not going to be true of me. Within a year of surgery my arms can extend and lift me to the top of a climbing wall; my lungs are strong enough to hike along mountain paths.

The same website concludes:

> Unfortunately, even though surgery can help reduce your symptoms, the cancer does return in many patients—regardless of whether part, or all, of the lung was removed. This is more likely in some patients than others, so you should talk with your healthcare providers about your particular situation. It's important that you and your doctor have the same expectations about the lobectomy.

But we don't. He still doesn't think I need a mammogram. I have a routine colonoscopy as a defiant vote for the need to think five years out. Some rebellion. Some detachment.

A Good Death

By the light of my silvery iPhone I softly sing my mother to her final sleep.

Kel and I have been with her for two weeks. We had originally planned to come stay with her while my sister, Annie, her husband, Doug, and daughter, Sarah, chaperone his middle school robotics team that has made it to the World Championship in Dallas. However, we caught an earlier flight as soon as we learned that my mother had been hospitalized for acute renal failure.

The hospital is like entering a dangerously upside-down parallel universe. Instead of hearing results of blood work within an hour, like I do at Seattle Cancer Care Alliance, it took four days before my mother's doctor read her labs and told her to check herself into the hospital. Instead of having Dr. Eaton play quarterback for any specialists involved in my care, my mother is passed from hospitalist to hospitalist, each one attacking only the most pressing issue of the day; none of them look at the whole problem.

"I don't like that doctor," is my mother's answer to the question of what ails her, and I remember how I, too, didn't like the surgeon who told me I was dying. But these doctors aren't that direct, never set a larger context, don't admit to being perplexed, and my mother rightfully perceives their tone as condescending. I finally draw a picture of my mother with arrows pointing to each distressed organ system, listing every symptom she exhibits and every test result we have, or is pending.

"That's a great diagram," says our fifth hospitalist. It's not about the drawing, it's about the woman before you, I think to myself. But he is the first to see the big picture. "It may be multiple myeloma, a cancer of the blood," he tells me out of my mother's hearing. "I'll start the tests, and we'll go from there."

Although death has been hovering around my door for four years, I have never been in the room with it. I have, in fact, been vigorously running away from it. Whereas I had determinedly walked lap after lap around the nurses' station after the lobectomy, my mother refuses to walk at all. While I had watched everything I ate, careful to get the fruits, vegetables, and protein I needed to heal, my mother refuses all food but yogurt and chocolate ice cream. While I had listened to every subtle signal of my body to help it back to health, if my mother is listening all she hears is a plea to get out of the hospital, ignore the doctor's orders, and return to the house she loves.

She goes home for three days. Instead of her normal four food groups—cookies, cake, chocolate, and ice cream—we struggle to get her to eat some protein and drink anything. But although she reads the Daily Beast online, watches Jon Stewart, and comments on the state of the world's financial crisis, when it comes to the subject of her own health crisis, she is mum, seemingly unable to calculate that if you don't eat, drink, or move, you die.

Back in the hospital, as her blood clots in her legs but leaks somewhere internally, she is told she has cancer by the sixth doctor, who not only breaks the news prematurely (we know there are two tests pending), but does it without grace and then abruptly leaves the room, never returning, and without having discussed any of Mom's treatment options.

"How do you feel about what the doctor just said, Mom?" I ask knowing how devastating this moment can be.

"We made a great decision today," she replies.

"What was that, Mom?"

She pauses. "I can't remember." More silence. "Oh, yes. Morphine." Yes, that is a good alternative to finding out you have cancer when you have no strength, or will, to acknowledge it, much less fight it. The team of doctors on duty, however, does try to fight it. A surgeon is brought in. "I could perform a colonoscopy to try to find the source of the internal bleeding." An oncologist is brought in. "We could start a protocol." But finally a new doctor, an angel in a white coat, looks at my mother's chart, with its record of system after system already closing down, observes my mother's failing strength, and asks my brother and me to join her in the waiting room. Tell me about your mother, she asks, as if she has come over for tea and we have all day. Tell me about yourselves and your sister. Tell me about your children.

Only after that does she say, "Although the results are still out from one blood test, your mother likely has multiple myeloma. It is a very demanding treatment protocol and I don't think she has the strength for it. Do you know what her wishes are? Does she have a Living Will?"

Finally we've found someone who has the courage and empathy to tell us the truth in a helpful way. My brother Cliff and I know exactly what my mother wants done. Pain relief. Nothing else. Her Living Will is explicit, and Cliff has recently re-read it to me. Over the years she has told us her wishes over and over, and she has done the same with my sister Annie. There is no ambiguity, no possibility of one sibling reading the situation differently from another. This is her gift to us.

"Then we will make her comfortable, and I don't think it will be long. When do Annie, Doug, and Sarah return from Texas?"

"Tomorrow night."

"Maybe they will make it in time."

The doctor walks back into Mom's room with us and gently tells her, "We are cancelling the colonoscopy and we are going to give you more morphine to make you comfortable. Is that what you want, to be comfortable?" My mother nods. Does she know the doctor has told her she is going to die soon, and that her last moments will be morphine-filled? Again, I ask my mom how she feels about what the doctor has said.

"I didn't like that nurse last night."

"That's no problem, Mom, we're moving you into your own private room, and the nurse won't be allowed in."

And so for the next thirty-eight hours, one of us always holds her hand. The doctor orders a hospitality cart filled with coffee and juice for us, and tells the nurses no one is to enter the room without our permission. No more random checks and hospital routines unless requested. My mother's death will be honored, instead of fitted into the hospital schedule. She passes quickly into unconsciousness while Kel, Cliff, and his wife and son, Carol and Calvin, talk with her, hold her, and do her prized *New York Times* Crossword Puzzle in her presence. My brother holds one hand and I the other, feeling our lifetime connection through our mother, returning in our hearts to the time when we were young and held her hand regularly.

At midnight, twenty-six hours since her last word or gesture, her eyes pop open.

"You're awake! We love you, Mom," we quickly say.

"I love you, too" are her last words. With nearly superhuman strength, she holds onto our hands, tries to pulls herself up, then lapses back into unconsciousness.

That night I sing her songs that were popular when she danced the night away at sock hops during the war. I search for lyrics of the top hits of the 1930s and 1940s, and work my way through the list. Mood Indigo. I'll Be Seeing You. When You Wish Upon a Star.

At 5:30 am, the nurses come in to bathe her and I leave the room to go down the hall to the restroom. A nurse quickly runs down the hall to find me. "Her breathing has fallen below 6 breaths per second. It's usually very quick now."

The angel doctor concurs, "Yes, it will be fast from now on. I'm afraid Annie will not make it."

The four of us start to improvise a ritual as my mother's breaths fall to 5 then 4 breaths per minute. We play her favorite symphonies. Annie, Doug, and Sarah join us on the phone to sing her favorite song, *What a Wonderful World,* to her. We manage between us to sing about one word in ten, and count on Israel Kamakawiwo'ole to sing the rest. Annie says her goodbyes over the phone. We leave the room to give Calvin, the only grandchild there, some time alone with my mother. But she holds on. At 11 am, five hours after the nurse first sounded the alarm, I realize that we can now reach all the grandchildren, including the three on the west coast.

"Would you like to say goodbye to Maman?"

Each in turn speaks words of love into her ear. I notice that Mom's gasping breathing appears to coincide with their pauses, as if she's consciously answering them. After all six grandchildren have their final moments, I email my mother's best friend. Immediately, I get a call from her.

"Yes, please put me through to your mother."

And after I click End Call, my mother's breathing goes back up to six breaths a minute and stays that way all afternoon. Around 5:30 pm, now twelve hours after death was supposedly imminent, we start to believe that not only can Mom make it until Annie arrives, but that she is waiting for her. We start telling her how long she has to wait. Just 3 more hours, Mom. Just two more. We do 4-on-1 Reiki, with Kelly at her head, me at her feet, and Cliff and Carol on each hand. It doesn't matter that Cliff has never tried Reiki. Hold on, Mom, hold on. When Annie, Doug and Sarah run into the hospital at 9:30, we are all exhilarated, punch-drunk that Mom has cared so much to wait. We say goodbye to her and go home for the night, leaving Annie and Doug to have the time alone with her that we've had. At 11:25 pm on April 25, my mother opens her eyes, looks at them, squeezes their hands, and dies.

I didn't know that love for your children and the strength of your will can underpin even your last moments. I didn't know our spirits were this powerful, even when our bodies have failed. My brother tells friends that she died "a good death." I hope I will be as lucky whenever my time comes. No pain, my loved ones at my side. There is a time to let go, and my mother timed hers perfectly.

April 7, 2010 — Clues

I don't know why I got cancer. I don't know whether I still have it. I don't know whether taking Tarceva is still necessary, or whether it's sufficient. I don't know whether the cancer will recur. This is simply life as I, and many cancer patients, know it.

Yet I am well. And this is enough to bring tears to my nurse's eyes as she reads my all-clear scans, one year after surgery. "I can't believe it. Seriously. I've never seen this." This is enough for Dr. Eaton to hug me when he walks in: "You've achieved a personal best." We have broken this cancer's cycle of forcing us to take new action every nine months. This is enough for Dr. Rockhill's new nurse to look at me with wonder.

Am I real? She looks at my color, posture, demeanor, reflexes, and energy; she listens to my lungs, heartbeat, and belly; she confirms that I can hear, focus, and point; she asks me to demonstrate that I can balance with my eyes closed, walk heel to toe, and push and pull against her hands. She asks me questions to see if I have any issues with all the systems in my body that the goddesses have cared for so well: respiration, heart, digestion, endocrine, skin, etc.

"Nope. Nope. Nope. Nope. Nope," I say, shaking my head. The nurse speeds up her questions before putting down her pad.

"You're in perfect health," she says, as if realizing that her questions only represent a three-dimensional map for the four-dimensional world she has just discovered.

Yes, I am. This is not just the absence of pain, malaise, depression, discomfort, coughing, headache, nausea, etc. This is the presence of well-being, strength, grace, joy, love. This is feeling great. To achieve this level of health, I've added another doctor to my team: I now meet individually with Dr. Sun for medical Qigong sessions. After his successful clinical trials testing the effectiveness of Qigong for the treatment of diabetes,[94] I have begun working with him in a study of Qigong and cancer. His method for evaluating my condition is to put both of his hands on either side of one of mine, a few inches away. From there he can read my energy flows—and with increasing accuracy, so can I.

He treats me by balancing the energy and boosting it, again with his hands in proximity to, but not touching, my body. With my eyes closed, I can tell which organ system he is working on because of the intense heat it generates in my body, like a forest fire clearing out old debris. (This effect may even be visible on CT scans. After a session strengthening my immune system, my thymus—the organ responsible for creating those warriors of the immune system, the T-cells—was, in the radiologist's words, "energized" on my CT scan three days later.) I recreate these sensations daily, strengthening the energy connections, until I see him again.

Dr. Sun also gives me specific ideas for where to focus my Qigong practice during the next month, never failing to encourage me. "You have been making great progress in your healing journey, and in developing greater awareness and internal strength." And he inspires me, too. "Moments of loss and death, awareness and enlightenment can be freeing moments, moments when you step away from the darkness in the box and walk away. However, you can also pull the darkness out the box and transform it into something that can be used to heal others." I am thrilled to have access to quality medical Qigong. I always leave our appointments feeling higher than a kite, and I never forget that the prime responsibility for healing lies with me, not my doctors.

So what am I doing now in my daily lab, now that I'm no longer working to keep cancer away, but to enhance my wellness? What do I do to keep my cells nourished, their waterworks clear, their software updated, their communication channels open, and their batteries charged? It's a simple list.

- I eat less, and eat well.
- I drink (tea and water) more often.
- I walk as much as I can.
- I keep my spirits lifted.
- I keep my energies charged.
- I listen to my inner world.
- I stay connected to my family, my friends, and the wondrous world we live in.
- I fill my heart with love and joy, and let it guide my way.
- I snuggle next to Kel at night, thankful for the day I've just lived.

Today Kelly has placed presents wrapped in cloth bags on the hearth to celebrate my 4th birthday. They are full of potential: a promise to travel the back roads of our own state, a journal to record our travels, and a book for when we come to rest. I just take in the sensation of being alive, and the joy of loving and being loved. I sit next to him by the fire, not moving, not reaching out for any present other than the one I'm in. I treasure all the people in my life who share my joy today. I am grateful for this body full of cells that feel so vibrantly alive.

Epilogue

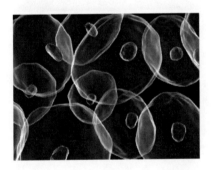

From: Diana and Kelly
Date: March 25, 2011
Subject: Thank you for 5 years and much much more

Dear amazing wonderful support team,

It has been nearly 5 years since you gathered around me physically or virtually to help me through stage IV lung cancer. At the time, my doctor said the odds of me writing to you now were 1%.

I just had my scans read yesterday and there is no evidence of cancer, in fact no evidence of any disease! And the only symptoms I'm experiencing from Tarceva are curly hair and long eyelashes. I am completely healthy and well. I asked the nurse, "If being alive at 5 years puts me in the 1% Club, what does this state of health put me in?" "Your own club," she answered.

Personally, I believe it's our club and that is why I am writing what I hope to be a final group email to thank you all for all the many surges of love, prayers, and energy you have sent us. We were probably all brought up with "it is more blessed to give than receive," so we shortchange our ability to receive. The Love-In shattered all that for me. At any moment afterward I could relive the feeling of so many of you encircling me. This got me through the Gamma Knife radiation.

It wasn't hard to imagine those hugs when you weren't there, and then to extend that to all those I have loved, regardless of space or time. When I would unpack the memory of what we meant to each other, I think I also unpacked the endorphins that went with those memories, giving me more healing power. I began to sense your presence when you weren't there—easy to do with email—but then I discovered I didn't need such primitive technology. During my CyberKnife radiation I felt you in the meadow, and you may remember the party we had afterwards, hugging, singing and dancing in a spirit-to- spirit network. It hasn't always been a party. You have also walked with me in the middle of the night when pain has overwhelmed me. You created a buoyant carpet for me to ride into the Surgery Pavilion, giving me the courage to keep going.

And somewhere along the way, you realized that you could call on me too. My oldest friend just fell off a cliff on the Na Pali Coast in Kauai while hiking before her daughter's wedding.

Very fortunately, a piece of her clothing caught on a ledge. While she waited on that ledge to be rescued, she realized she had the choice while she was there to panic or be calm. "I went to the meadow," she called to tell me. "Wasn't it wonderful?" I asked her. "What happened there?" "Well, everyone picked me up and carried me everywhere," she replied. And that's the way it has been for me these past five years, too—and could be for you anytime you need it.

You are an amazing group of people. You have founded companies, funded them, managed them, worked in them, rescued them, and retired from them. You are healers of all sorts—surgeons, doctors, PAs, ARPNs, dentists, nurses, therapists, acupuncturists, chiropractors, massage therapists, energy healers (even lawyers). You are teachers of the young and old, and lifelong students. You create with your bodies as carpenters, dancers, and farmers, with your minds as writers, choreographers, composers, architects, and artists, and with others as producers, directors, and managers. The term 501(c)(3) trips off your tongue: you create non-profits, volunteer your time, and contribute financially. You are single, married, divorced, and widowed. You have children, grandchildren, and great grand-children, and have chosen not to have any of the above. Most of you know me, but some of you I have never met. You have taken all this skill and talent that you have spent a lifetime build-ing and out of the goodness of your heart and soul applied it in many varied ways to my healing—forms of Fate Management that you may or may not have been comfortable with.

We did it! Who would have thought it possible? Share our story to give others hope when they need it.

With much love and gratitude,
Diana and Kelly

Thea, Jasper, and I are walking hand in hand to the park after having picked up Thea from kindergarten. Pink and orange-flowered backpack bobbing on her back, Thea tells me about her day.

"Do you know about the buckets, Nin?" she asks.

"No, tell me about them, Thea."

"Well, everyone has one, but they're invisible," she whispers conspiratorially. "They are filled with all the nice things in your life. If someone does something mean to you, they take something from your bucket."

"Has this ever happened to you, Thea?"

"Yes." And she tells me briefly about a boy at recess, but this is not the point of her story. "But if you do something nice for someone, you fill up their bucket and you fill up your own."

"Have you tried that, Thea? Did it work that way?"

"Yes, I helped my friend, Richard, and then I felt better too."

"You always fill my bucket, Thea. You're a bucket-filler."

"When we're together, our buckets are always full, Nin."

Acknowledgements

My first (and forever) thanks goes to family: to those near who surrounded me immediately with their love—Susan, Tom, Jessie, John, Jake—and to those who arrived quickly—Targe, Joanne, Nancy, Tim, Siena, Targe, Barb, David, Kristina, Anne, Doug, Sabina, Sarah, Cliff, Carol, Calvin, and Ted.

My gratitude to all of those at Lindsay Communications and Daves & Associates, especially Nancy Daves, Monica Uhl, and Linda Schaefer who gave me the flexibility to devote my time to healing.

A community of hundreds from near and far joined me in the Joy Protocol, but special thanks to Rene, Miles, Randy, Georgia, Doug, Dana, Bob, Bonnie, Steve, Debora, Kären, Bob, Lynn, Ellen, Craig, and the Rural Characters for their devotion.

I have unending gratitude for the brilliance of my medical team: to oncologists Keith Eaton and Renato Martins, radiation oncologists Jason Rockhill and Vivek Mehta, surgeon Michael Mulligan, and all of their compassionate ARPNs but especially Leslie Anderson, Susan Treharne, and Sarah Layman. My integrative medical team was equally wise and deeply compassionate (in order of when I worked with them): Jin Shin Jyutsu practitioner April Lanz; massage practitioner Jill Clark on Whidbey Island and Victoria Bledsoe in Bloomington IN; chiropractor Robert Sleight; acupuncturist Tim Batiste; and physical therapist Shannon Arndt, all of whom are gifted healers with deep insight into the human psyche and body. I'd like to especially thank Dr. Guan-Cheng Sun for both the gift of his Yi Ren Qigong teaching and the astonishing strength of his energetic work with me as a medical Qigong practitioner and to Sarri Gilman who first taught me how to access and trust my inner wisdom.

I'd like to thank the researchers who furthered my understanding of cancer's biological processes and how they might correlate with my imagery: Dr. Gregory Holt, Dr. William Parks and all of the researchers at the University of Washington and National Institutes of Health who continue to study my genetics and response to genetic testing, blood, and tissue.

I'd also like to thank those who helped me turn my personal experience into a book for others: to Elizabeth George for listening to my story and thinking it was worth writing; to Peter Guzzardi, our editor, who brought his decades of brilliant talent to the shaping and smoothing of the story's arc and lines; and to Anne Edelstein, our agent, who not only believed in the story but contributed her own wisdom in presenting it. I'd like to thank our wonderful early readers and believers who helped us clarify our ideas: Tandy Beal, Doug and Dana Kelly, Susanne Fest, Roberta Bristol, Mary McKenna, Rick Ingrasci, Peggy Taylor, and Jerry Millhon. And thanks to Morgan Bondelid for her gift of design.

What has filled every moment of my eight years with cancer is my never-ending love for our children, Camilla and Isaac and Eric and Kylie, and our grandchildren, Thea, Jasper, Aidan, Eli, and Lena whose loving spirits fill my heart to bursting. But my deepest gratitude and love goes to Kelly who transformed his love into healing power and saved me.

Notes

CHAPTER ONE

[1] Sharon Begley, "What You Don't Know Might Kill You", *Newsweek*, October 17, 2009.

[2] Jill Bolte Taylor, *My Stroke of Insight,* (New York: Viking, 2006), 146.

[3] Mark Fischetti, "The Great Chemical Unknown: Only a tiny fraction of the compounds around us have been tested for safety", *Scientific American,* November 2010, 92.

[4] Smoking is also a contributing factor in 4 out of the top 5 causes of death according to the U.S. Centers for Disease Control and Prevention, "Final data, Leading Causes of Death 2007, Table B" from the *National Vital Statistics Report,* vol 58:19.

[5] Dr. Heather Wakelee, associate professor Stanford Cancer Center in a webinar presentation, "Never-Smokers and Gender Differences in Lung Cancer" based on her research: "Lung Cancer Incidence in Never Smokers", *Journal of Clinical Oncology,* Vol 25, No 5 (February 10, 2007): 472–478, doi: 10.1200/JCO.2006.07.2983

[6] "Erlotinib (Tarceva®) Extends Survival in Advanced Lung Cancer", Clinical Trial Results, National Cancer Institute, posted 6/05/2004. *http://www.cancer.gov/clinicaltrials/results/summary/2004/lung-and-erlotinib0604*

[7] "Tarceva nearly doubled the time people with a genetically distinct type of lung cancer lived without their disease getting worse", *www.roche.com,* accessed June 3, 2011.

[8] Chart notes from 5/4/2006 appointment with Dr. Jason Rockhill, Gamma Knife Center, Harborview Medical Center, Seattle WA.

CHAPTER TWO

[9] Andrew Weil, *Spontaneous Healing,* (NY: Fawcett Columbine Books, 1995), 37.

[10] Ibid., 75–76.

[11] Ibid., 83.

[12] Center for Disease Control and Prevention, National Program of Cancer Registries. United States Cancer Statistics. "1995–2005 Cancer Incidence and Mortality Data." *http://apps.nccd.cdc.gov/uscs/*

[13] National Cancer Institute, Surveillance, Epidemiology, and End Results database, based on people who were diagnosed with non-small cell lung cancer between 1998 and 2000 as cited by the American Cancer Society.

[14] "FDA Approves New Drug for the Most Common Type of Lung Cancer Drug Shows Survival Benefit," FDA News Release, P04-105, November 19, 2004.

[15] H. K. Beecher, "The Powerful Placebo," *Journal of the American Medical Association,* 1955;159(17):1602-1606. doi:10.1001/jama.1955.02960340022006.

[16] There are many sources if you'd like to explore the placebo effect further. Dr. Weil's work and Dr. Groopman's were most influential for me at this stage in my treatment. See Jerome Groopman, *The Anatomy of Hope,* (NY: Random House, 2004), p 168. For a discussion on the nocebo effect, see his note on p 229 based on work by Barsky, A., R. Saintfort, et al, "Nonspecific Medication Side Effects and the Nocebo Phenomenon," *The Journal of the American Medical Association,* 287 (2002): 622–627. More recent work includes Wells, R, Kaptchuk TJ., "To tell the truth, the whole truth, may do patients harm: The problem of the nocebo effect for informed consent." *The American Journal of Bioethics* 2012; 12(3): 22–29 and Finniss DG, Kaptchuk TJ, Miller F, Benedetti F., "Biological, clinical, and ethical advances of placebo effects.", *Lancet.* 2010 Feb 20; 375 (9715): 686-95.

[17] Citing research by Dr. Fabrizio Benedetti, Dept of Neuroscience at the University of Turin in Italy, Jerome Groopman wrote "Belief and expectation, cardinal components of hope, can block pain by releasing the brain's endorphins and enkephalins, thereby mimicking the effects of morphine" in his book *The Anatomy of Hope: How People Prevail in the Face of Illness* (NY: Random House, 2004), 170. Groopman cites J. Wybran's paper: "Enkephalins and endorphins as modifiers of the immune system: present and future" *Fed Proc.* 1985 Jan; 44(1 Pt 1):92-4.

[18] HostDefense mushrooms are currently marketed as MyCommunity mushrooms. See *http://www.fungi.com/supplements/capsules.html* for more information. For a full list of studies on the anti-cancer activity of medicinal mushrooms, read Paul Stamets, *MycoMedicinals: An Informational Treatise on Mushrooms,* (Olympia: MycoMedia Productions, 2002).

[19] There have been many studies of the importance of support in cancer survival dating from a 1989 study at Stanford University by David Spiegel that showed group therapy improved survival time in metastatic breast cancer patients. I heard Professor Spiegel speak about his study at the time and it made a big impression on me. A more recent study is by Ann F. Chou, Susan L. Stewart, Robert C. Wild, Joan R. Bloom, "Social support and survival in young women with breast carcinoma", *Pscho-Oncology,* published online Oct 20, 2010. doi: 10.1002/pon.1863

[20] Radiologyinfo.org, accessed September 28, 2009, *http://www.radiologyinfo.org/en/info.cfm?pg=gamma_knife*

21 Daniel Pink, *A Whole New Mind,* (NY: Riverhead Books, 2005), 26.

22 Although my knowledge of the Simonton work was only through a vague memory of 1980s press stories about how visualizing the cancer fight can impact survival, the Simonton Cancer Center is still active. Check out *www.simontoncenter.com* for more information. *Getting Well Again* is Dr. Carl Simonton's most known book.

23 *http://www.candacepert.com/,* accessed on February 17, 2010.

24 Research by Harvard neuroscientist Gottfried Schlaug has shown that the front portion of the corpus callosum, the fiber highway between the two hemispheres of the brain, is larger in musicians than non-musicians. See Gaser, Cl, and G. Schlaug, "Gray matter differences between musicians and nonmusicians", *Annals of the New York Academy of Sciences,* 999:514–517 (2003).

25 Daniel Levitin, *The World in Six Songs,* (NY: Dutton, 2008), 92.

26 Belle Waring, "Goosebumps in G Major: Levitin Reveals Your Brain on Music", *nih record, http://nihrecord.od.nih.gov/newsletters/2008/03_21_2008/story3.htm*

CHAPTER THREE

27 Thomas, Lewis, *The Medusa and the Snail: More Notes of a Biology Watcher,* (NY: Viking Press, 1979), 30.

28 The benefits of outdoor exercise include higher Vitamin D levels, elevated mood, and faster healing according to "A prescription for better health: Go alfresco", *Harvard HealthBeat* newsletter, October 12, 2010.

29 Sandra Blakeslee, "Cells that Read Minds", *The New York Times,* January 10, 2006.

30 A 2010 study by the National Center for Complementary and Alternative Medicine, a division of the National Institute of Health, found a single session of deep touch massage significantly decreases the stress hormone cortisol and increases the number of lymphocytes which are part of the immune system. Mark Hyman Rapaport, Pamela Schettler, Catherine Bresee, "A Preliminary Study of the Effects of a Single Session of Swedish Massage on Hypothalamic–Pituitary–Adrenal and Immune Function in Normal Individuals" *The Journal of Alternative and Complementary Medicine.* October 2010, 16(10): 1079–1088. PMID: 20809811

31 "A new study has revealed for the first time how kneading eases sore muscles— by turning off genes associated with inflammation and turning on genes that help muscles heal" wrote Gisela Telis, "Massage's Mystery Mechanism Unmasked", *Science Now,* February 1, 2012, reporting on a study by Mark Tarnopolsky, a neurometabolic researcher at McMaster University in Hamilton, Canada published in *Science Translational Medicine,* February 2012.

32 USGS, "Science for a Changing world, The Water in You" *http://ga.water.usgs.gov/edu/propertyyou.html*

33 Deane Juhan, *Job's Body,* (NY: Station Hill Openings, 1998), 59.

[34] While daydreaming connotes pleasant thoughts, in the article "When the Mind Wanders Happiness Also Strays", John Tierney (*The New York Times*, November 15, 2010) cites researchers Matthew Killingsworth and Daniel Gilbert as saying "When people (mind) wander, they are just as likely to wander toward negative thoughts." Their study also showed minds of their subjects were wandering 47 percent of the time.

[35] "Brain Waves and Meditation", *ScienceDaily* (Mar. 31, 2010) Professor Jim Lagopoulos of Sydney University, Australia. Lagopoulos is the principal investigator of a joint study between his university and researchers from the Norwegian University of Science and Technology (NTNU) on changes in electrical brain activity during nondirective meditation. During meditation, theta waves were most abundant in the frontal and middle parts of the brain. "These types of waves likely originate from a relaxed attention that monitors our inner experiences. Here lies a significant difference between meditation and relaxing without any specific technique," emphasizes Lagopoulos. "Previous studies have shown that theta waves indicate deep relaxation and occur more frequently in highly experienced meditation practitioners. The source is probably frontal parts of the brain, which are associated with monitoring of other mental processes."

CHAPTER FOUR

[36] Andrew Weil, *Breathing: The Master Key to Self Healing* CD (Sounds True, Incorporated, 1999.)

[37] Liz Szabo, "Certain Cells are More Lethal", *USA TODAY*, February 26, 2007.

CHAPTER FIVE

[38] Malcolm Gladwell, *Blink: The Power of Thinking Without Thinking,* (N.Y.: Little, Brown and Company, 2005), 34.

[39] Mary R. Kwaan, MD, MPH; David M. Studdert, LLB, ScD; Michael J. Zinner, MD; Atul A. Gawande, MD, "MPH Incidence, Patterns, and Prevention of Wrong-Site Surgery", *Archives of Surgery*, Vol 141, April 2006.

[40] Dr. Mehta's chart notes, 9/5/07 appointment.

[41] Nora Isaacs, "Exercisers Slow It Down With Qigong", *The New York Times,* April 5, 2007.

[42] By 2010, researchers would begin to capture this electricity for body-powered devices. "Everything we do generates power—about 1 watt per breath, 70 watts per step." "The 50 Best Inventions of the Year 2010: Body-Powered Devices," *Time*, November 22, 2010, 88.

CHAPTER SIX

[43] Living With Uncertainty: The Fear of Cancer Recurrence, American Cancer Society, *http://www.cancer.org/acs/groups/cid/documents/webcontent/002014-pdf.pdf*

[44] Ray Long MD FRCSC, *The Key Muscles of Hatha Yoga*, (Bandha Yoga Publications, 2005), 10.

[45] Wheway J., Herzog H., and Mackay F. "The Role of Neuropeptide Y and its Receptors in the Immune System and Immune Disorders, NPY and receptors in immune and inflammatory diseases", *Current Topics in Medicinal Chemistry.* 2007;7(17):1743–52. "At the Garvan Institute, we recently discovered that neuropeptide Y (NPY), a hormone secreted during psychological stress, interferes with immune defenses and inhibits the response of important immune cells via the Y1 receptor. This was an important discovery as, for the first time, we established a new link between psychological stress and immuno-suppression." Wheway J., Herzog H., and Mackay F. "The Y1 receptor for NPY: a key modulator of the adaptive immune system", *Peptides.* 2007 Feb;28(2):453–8.

[46] S. C. Vaughan, *The Talking Cure: The Science Behind Psychotherapy.* (New York: Grosset/Putnam, 1997).

[47] Norman Doidge, *The Brain that Changes Itself: Stories of Personal Triumph from the Frontiers of Brain Science,* (London: Penguin Books, 2007), 117.

[48] Edge 116, May 19, 2003, "In the Matrix: Martin Rees", *http://www.edge.org/documents/archive/edge116.html*

[49] James Plummer, Terman Dean of the School of Engineering, Stanford University during a speech at the Stanford symposium: Leading Matters, Seattle, January 26, 2008.

[50] Daniel Gilbert, *Stumbling on Happiness,* (NY: Knopf, 2006), 238.

[51] Gregory Cochran, "There is something new under the sun—us" *What is your dangerous idea?* The World Question Center, accessed on *edge.com* in 2006, *http://edge.org/response-detail/10750*

[52] Sam Schechner, "Keeping Love Alive: Neuroscientists are probing why some married couples can maintain the spark for years", *Wall Street Journal,* February 8, 2008, W1. For more information see H. E. Fisher, L. L. Brown, A. Aron, G. Strong, D. Mashek. "Reward, Addiction and Emotion Regulation Systems Associated with Rejection in Love". *Journal of Neurophysiology,* 2010; DOI: 10.1152/jn.00784.2009.

[53] Louann Brizendine, M.D. *The Female Brain,* (Broadway books, 2006), 105.

[54] Basus, Dasupta PS, "Dopamine, a neurotransmitter, influences the immune system". *Journal of Neuroimmunology,* 2000 Jan 24; 102 (2): 113–24, and Heinrichs M, Baumgartner T, Kirschbaum C, Ehlert U, "Social support and oxytocin interact to suppress cortisol and subjective responses to psychological stress". *Biol Psychiatry,* 2003;54:1389–1398.

[55] Doidge, M.D., op. cit., 120.

[56] "There is a two-week window, or critical period, about a month after these new cells hatch during which they act like the neurons of a newborn baby. During this time, the cell synapses (connections that allow neurons to communicate with each other) that are artificially stimulated become stronger. This strengthening results in more efficient information transmission between cells, and is thought to prime them to learn," according to Nikhil Swaminathan. "New Neurons in Old Brains Exhibit Babylike Plasticity", *Scientific American*, May 23, 2007, *http://www.scientificamerican.com/article/new-neurons-in-old-brains/*

[57] Ibid.

[58] Ibid.

[59] Dr. Luciano Bernardi of the University of Padua demonstrated that "…all the different biological rhythms being measured started to resonate, mutually amplifying each other to create a smooth, harmonious pattern" that he called coherence when a congregation recited a rosary or a Buddhist mantra. (Bernardi, L., P. Sleight, G. Bandinelli, et al., "Effect of Rosary Prayer and Yoga mantras on Autonomic Cardiovascular Rhythms: Comparative study," *British Medical Journal* 323 (2001): 1446–49. This state of coherence results in better functioning of the immune system according to Julian Thayer and Esther Sternberg, National Institutes of Health, Annals of the New York Academy of Sciences, quoted in David Servan-Shreiber, *Anti-cancer*, (NY; Viking, 2008), 160.

[60] Swaminathan, op. cit.

[61] Doidge, M.D., op. cit., 114.

[62] Deepak Chopra, *Journey into Healing, Awakening the Wisdom Within You*, (NY: Harmony Books, 1994), 32.

[63] Jill Bolte Taylor, TED talk filmed February 2008: *http://www.ted.com/talks/ jill_bolte_taylor_s_powerful_stroke_of_insight.html*

[64] Stephen S Hall, "Revolution Postponed", *Scientific American*, October 2010, 60.

[65] Genentech website, June 1, 2010, "Q&A: Genentech's Zemin Zhang on Whole-Genome Sequencing of Lung Cancer Samples", *http://www.genomeweb.com/sequencing/ qa-genentechs-zemin-zhang-whole-genome-sequencing-lung-cancer-samples*

[66] Laura Beil, "Medicine's New Epicenter? Epigenetics", *Cure*, Winter 2008, 37.

[67] Wikipedia website, accessed 2010, *http://en.wikipedia.org/wiki/Epigenetics*

[68] "The brain evolved watching music and listening to it at the same time. When we hear music our motor cortex fires up, so to keep still, we have to suppress it," said Daniel Levitin as quoted by Belle Waring, "Goosebumps in G Major: Levitin Reveals Your Brain on Music", *NIH Record*, Vol. LX, No. 8, March 21, 2008. Research by HeartMath found that the combination of music and meditation increased IgA levels (an immune system marker) by 141 percent, Doc Childre and Howard Martin, *The HeartMath Solution*, (SF: HarperSanFrancisco, 1999), 221.

[69] David Freedman, "The Streetlight Effect", *Discover Magazine*, July/August 2010, 55. A summary of his book *Wrong* (NY: Little, Brown, 2010).

70 Joan O'Connell Hamilton, "Something doesn't add up", *Stanford Magazine*, May/June 2012.

71 Freedman, op.cit., 56.

72 Andrew Pollak ,"Forty Years' War For Profit, Industry Seeks Cancer Drugs", *The New York Times*, September 1, 2009.

73 Sanjaya Kumar and David B. Nash, "Health Care Myth Busters: Is There a High Degree of Scientific Certainty in Modern Medicine? Two doctors take on the health care system in a new book that aims to arm people with information", *Scientific American*, March 25, 2011.

CHAPTER SEVEN

74 These mental loops are simplified, meditative versions of the Yi-Ren Qigong practice developed by Dr. Guang-Chen Sun. See *www.iqim.org* for more information. Used with permission.

75 David Servan-Shreiber, *Anti-cancer*, (NY; Viking, 2008).

CHAPTER EIGHT

76 John Ding, E Young , Chau-Ching Lin, and Gilla Kaplan, "Cytotoxic Lymphocyte Destroying a Tumor Cell", ASM MicrobeLibrary.org.

77 Carol A. de la Motte, "Mononuclear Leukocytes Bing to Specific Hyaluronan Structures on Colon Mucosal Smooth Muscle Cells Treated with Polyinosinic Acid", *The American Journal of Pathology*, vol. 163 (2003), 121.

78 Woods JA, Davis JM. Department of Exercise Science, School of Public Health, University of South Carolina, Columbia "Exercise, monocyte/macrophage function, and cancer". 29208. *Medicine & Science in Sports & Exercise*. 1994 Feb 26(2):147–56.

79 Robert P Mecham and John Heuser "The Elastic Fiber" chapter 3 of *Cell biology of extracellular matrix* ed. Elizabeth D. Hay, (NY: Plenum Press, 1991), 95 figure 3-8. With kind permission from Springer Science and Business Media.

80 Ibid, 94.

81 "Lung Cancer Cells Activate Inflammation To Induce Metastasis", *NewsRx.com*, January 15, 2009 reporting research by Michael Karin, Ph.D., in *Nature*.

82 Reginald F. Munden, Kenneth R. Hess. "Ditzels" on Chest CT: Survey of Members of the Society of Thoracic Radiology, *http://www.ajronline.org/cgi/reprint/176/6/1363.pdf*

83 Lee F. Rogers, "Ditzels: Little Things Mean A Lot", *American Journal of Roentgenology*, 2001 176:6, 1355-1355 *http://www.ajronline.org/doi/abs/10.2214/ajr.176.6.1761355*

[84] In May 2009, within a few months of our session, University of Montreal scientists published a paper in the *International Journal of Cancer* linking lung cancer with women whose menopause had been induced medically as mine had when I had a total hysterectomy and went off estrogen fairly abruptly following reports of the dangers of hormone replacement therapy. Koushik, A., Parent, M.-É. and Siemiatycki, J. (2009), "Characteristics of menstruation and pregnancy and the risk of lung cancer in women". *International Journal of Cancer*, 125: 2428–2433.

[85] Stephen M. Rappaport and Martyn T. Smith, "Environment and Disease Risks", *Science*, 22 Vol. 330: 6003. 460–461.

[86] Laura Beil, "Medicine's New Epicenter? Epigenetics", *Cure*, Winter 2008, 43.

[87] NIH website, "Human Cells 101", *http://www.nichd.nih.gov/publications/pubs/fragileX/sub3.cfm*

[88] Carl J. Charnetski and Francis X. Brennan, (2004) "Sexual Frequency and Salivary Immunoglobulin A (IgA)". *Psychological Reports:* Volume 94, June , 839–844. PMID: 15217036

CHAPTER TEN

[89] Carly Simon/Jacob Brackman, "Haven't got time for the pain".

[90] Jerry Lopper, "Relieve Pain With Mindpower: Stanford University research says to reduce pain focus attention elsewhere, perceive the pain as weak, and see soothing images", *suite101.com*, Aug 23, 2006, citing research by R. Christopher deCharms et al, "Control over brain activation and pain learned by using real-time functional MRI", *PNAS*, August 21, 2012, 109 (34).

[91] The stretching institute website, *http://www.thestretchinghandbook.com/archives/scar-tissue.php*

[92] In the 4/14/10 issue of *The New York Times*, I will read research by James Coan of the University of Virginia who found that a happily married woman who held her husband's hand calmed the brain regions associated with pain just like a pain-relieving drug in the article "Is Marriage Good for Your Health?" by Tara Parker-Pope. She quotes Coan: "When someone holds your hand in a study or just shows that they are there for you by giving you a back rub, when you're in their presence, that becomes a cue that you don't have to regulate your negative emotion. The other person is essentially regulating your negative emotion but without your prefrontal cortex. It's much less wear and tear on us if we have someone there to help regulate us."

[93] emedtv website, accessed 2009, *http://lung-cancer.emedtv.com/lobectomy/lobectomy-expectations.html*

[94] Sun GC, Lovejoy J, Gillham S, Putiri A, Sasagawa M, and Bradley R. "The Effects of Qigong on Glucose Control in Type 2 Diabetes: A Randomized Controlled Pilot Study". *Diabetes Care*, 2010. 33(1):e8. PMID: 20040671.

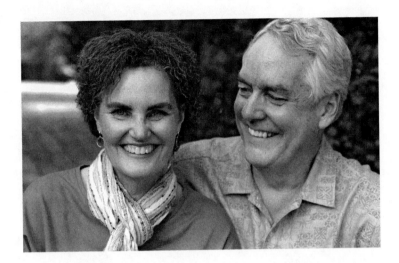

About the Authors

Diana and Kelly Lindsay were co-owners of Lindsay Communications, a strategic marketing consulting company when Diana was diagnosed with terminal cancer in 2006. Today they inspire patients, caregivers, researchers, and the general public to find something more than hope in the face of crisis. They teach Body/Mind Healing for Antioch University and are the founders of *Healing Circles Langley* on Whidbey Island, WA.

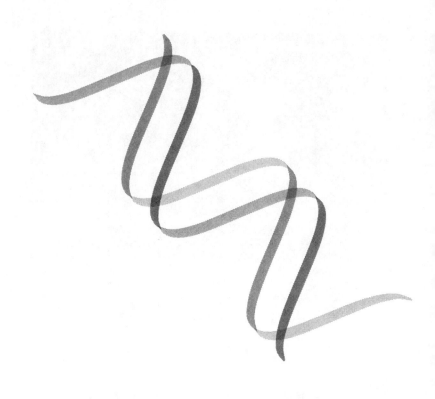

*To follow Diana and Kelly's continuing stories,
or to ignite your own healing power with tips and tools,
please visit somethingmorethanhope.com*

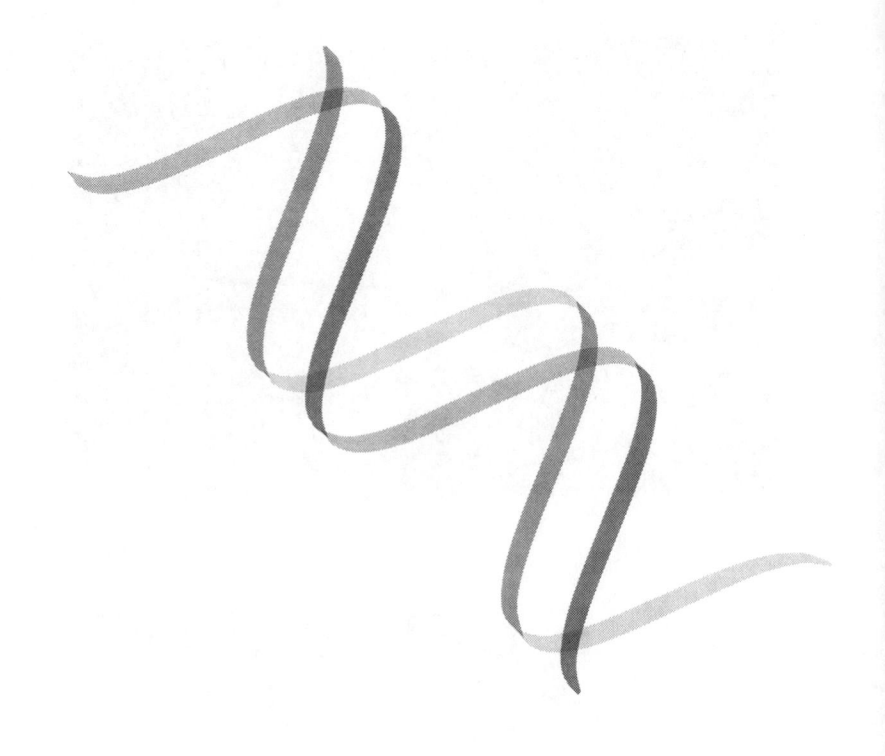

To follow Diana and Kelly's continuing stories,
or to ignite your own healing power with tips and tools,
please visit somethingmorethanhope.com

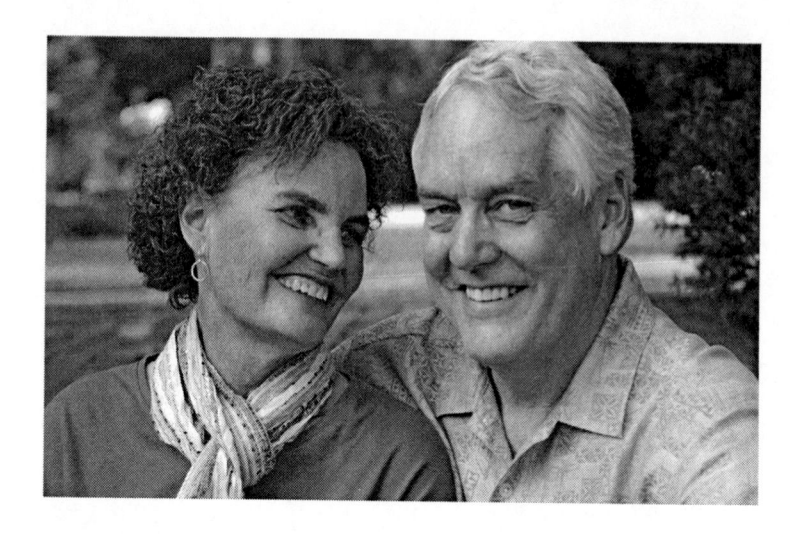

About the Authors

Diana and Kelly Lindsay were co-owners of Lindsay Communications, a strategic marketing consulting company, when Diana was diagnosed with terminal cancer in 2006. Today they inspire patients, caregivers, researchers, and the general public to find something more than hope in the face of crisis. They teach Body/Mind Healing for Antioch University and are the founders of *Healing Circles Langley* on Whidbey Island, WA.

I would be remiss if I didn't thank the person who made this bizarre roadtrip possible. I have always been awestruck that Diana came into my life 40 years ago. I am grateful for who she is, has been, has become, and will be. I am especially thankful that she's still here, but I am even more thankful for the cancer that almost made her not here because that has pointed out to me what I'm most grateful for above all, and that is that the universe doesn't work as I would have it. It's much more marvelous than that.

CPSIA information can be obtained
at www.ICGtesting.com
Printed in the USA
FSOW01n0422280717
36693FS

9 780991 242702

"Diana and Kelly Lindsay have written a remarkable account of Diana's exceptional recovery from stage 4 lung cancer. They faced daunting odds with fierce intentionality and a wise integration of conventional and integrative therapies. Above all, they understand the healing power of love. A beautiful story, well told."

— Michael Lerner, President and Founder, Commonweal

"Diana and Kelly's moving journeys in the face of cancer affirm that miracles are made — not with blueprints or instruction manuals, but with courage, intuition, intelligence and abiding love. The honesty, humor and insights embedded in each chapter are unique to them as patient and caretaker, wife and husband, yet universal in their depiction of the human heart as it opens and closes and opens again to the onslaught of life in all its rawness and beauty. For those with a life-threatening illness and their loved ones, this book is like a dear friend at your side, reminding you that you are not alone, whatever your path may be."

— Elise Miller, MEd
Director, Collaborative on Health
and the Environment

"We read the book to each other and shared all the emotional ups and downs, visions and hopes that your story triggered in our minds. Both Diana and Kelly were able to express the fears, regrets, and questions that we were afraid to express to ourselves and to each other. Thank you so much for the hope you have given us! You don't know how your words have opened our hearts to face this new life with determination and a clear goal."

— Sara Giswold, caregiver of spouse newly
diagnosed with stage 4 ductal carcinoma

Something More Than Everything

Something More Than Than Everything

A caregiver's commentary on what went right when life went wrong

Kelly Lindsay

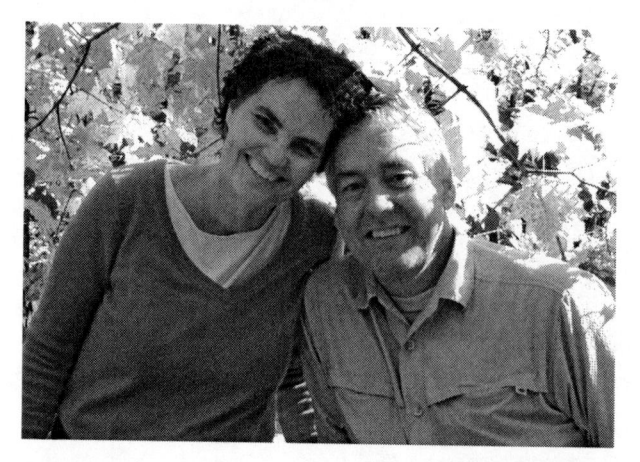

Inroads Press

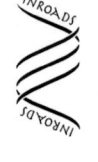

Inroads Press
P.O. Box 1308
534 Camano Avenue
Langley, WA 98260
inroadspress.com

The authors are grateful for use of the following copyrighted material:

The photographs are by permission of Diana & Kelly Lindsay with the following exceptions:

Tandy Beal & Company for photographs from the production of *HereAfterHere*. Photographs by Chunyi McIver.

Royalty-free stock images by Sebastian Kaulitzki (*dreamstime.com*).

Creative Commons photographs by Shane Porter.

Image reprinted from *The American Journal of Pathology,* vol. 163, Carol A. de la Motte, "Mononuclear Leukocytes Bing to Specific Hyaluronan Structures on Colon Mucosal Smooth Muscle Cells Treated with Polyinosinic Acid", page 121, copyright 2003, with permission from Elsevier.

Images reprinted from *Cell biology of the Extracellular Matrix,* ed. Elizabeth D. Hay, (NY: Plenum Press, 1991). With kind permission from Springer Science and Business Media.

Book design by Morgan Bondelid

Printed in the United States of America

ISBN 978-0-9912427-0-2

For our grandchildren

Table of Contents

Authors' Foreword

Sixteen minutes is the average lead time we get from a tornado warning. Just sixteen minutes to race to your children or grandchildren, grab them under your arm, and run to the nearest shelter. There isn't, however, an average recovery time. How long before we emerge from the shelter, stand on the ruin of a former home, and rebuild a life is up to us. It takes about four seconds to hear the words "You have cancer", "I want a divorce", or "I'm sorry for your loss." The rubble at your feet may not be shattered glass and splintered wood, but the devastation feels comparable.

The brain has difficulty handling these moments of utter vulnerability. Our common understandings of the world and habitual responses rip away like roof shingles in a 200 mile-per-hour wind. We might sob with anguish or stare blankly, but in that moment we are usually incapable of taking in anything else. And yet, most of us recover. Brain circuits reboot and begin processing again. We look around, sense a direction, and take a step forward. We are hardwired for resilience.

When we were told Diana had a terminal illness, at first we didn't believe there could be any way we could survive the blow. When Diana decided to pick up and start moving, our expectations were minimal. We had no way of knowing that the trek would revitalize our marriage, transform how we live and love, and deeply connect us to healing sources within us and in the world at large. We didn't yet have the imagination to conceive of a Love-In, a Gratitude Tour, a Cuddle Shuttle, or Skyping Diana's cells—much less acknowledge

them as messengers of healing.

We didn't have a clue that we would benefit along the way from Western medicine's latest advances in destroying cancer cells and Eastern energy medicine's guidance on strengthening our healthy cells. It was precisely the extreme narrowing of Diana's treatment options that forced us to expand our thinking enough to discover how to make our own medicine. It was only after losing the comfort of any familiar path that she discovered her body could guide her through the unknown.

If you've begun to read at this point, from here to the middle of the book you'll find Kelly's perspective on the same story, about giving up—and getting back—*Something More Than Everything* in his role as Diana's primary caregiver. Starting from the opposite end of the book you'll find Diana's story. It's about what happens when life both demands—and offers—*Something More Than Hope*. If you find yourself facing illness, catastrophe, or despair, we hope our story will ease your way as you find your own.

This book is not only about cancer. There are many moments in life when we are thrust into a bear pit that seems to have no way out but through the bear. It is not even about coming to a happy ending. It's about the hope and creativity, love and joy, awe and gratitude that come from drinking in every moment we're alive—no matter how many days we have left.

Something More Than Everything

Something more than everything

In April 2006, my wife of 31 years and a lifelong non-smoker was diagnosed with incurable Stage IV lung cancer and given 3 to 12 months to live. We are now just beyond the 8-year mark and she has no evidence of disease.

How is that possible, you might ask? That's a reasonable question, and there may even be a reasonable answer, but it's not really my place to give it. I'm not even sure it's my place to know it, especially since I find the whole idea of "knowing" somewhat suspect these days. What I *do* know—now—is that "How is that possible?" isn't really the right question, and the closest I could come to answering it is with another question: "Why wouldn't it be?"

Not long ago, Diana asked which I would choose if I could travel in time back to 2006: Door #1, with life continuing on as it had been, or Door #2, with the life we've had since. I didn't hesitate—and neither did she—in choosing Door #2.

For whatever it's worth, what follows is commentary on my role as the primary caregiver. This is not a how-to guide. It is also not exclusive to caregiving. I think life offers many opportunities or occasions that demand more than we want to give, more than we think we have in us to give. I was lucky. Diana had received a death sentence, and by extension, so had I. After getting over the initial shock, when I was tempted to give up altogether, it became a fairly straightforward negotiation: What could we trade that might

be worth two lives? Not in the long term, but today.

The following pages describe those exchanges. At first I thought we were in the position of *losing* everything. But I discovered that we could opt for *letting go* of everything instead, and—implausibly—get something more than that in return.

End of the world

Y ou don't come to the end of the world; the end of the world comes to you. You might see it coming; then again, you might not. I didn't.

When Diana was diagnosed with Stage IV lung cancer in 2006 and given months to live, the vanishing horizon of our future was no longer way out there; it approached at unimaginable speed, until it felt like I was waist-deep in freezing water peering into the proverbial void. But in fact, there wasn't anything there to see. I'd thought I could at least imagine the end of the world, but it was just nothingness. So I leaned into it, and fell.

Physicists have theorized the existence of black holes for some time now, and have debated what happens if you have the misfortune to approach one. There's some mention of unrelenting gravity that would crush you into an infinitely dense mass the size of a pinhead, with nothing for company but 40 dancing angels. But physicists have also theorized the existence of parallel universes, and the possibility that black holes may actually create "wormholes" that provide toll-free access from one universe to another. Now that kind of black hole was appealing. A different universe sounded good because this one was looking dismal. I needed a wormhole. Better yet, a rabbit hole.

At first I only saw a single, devastatingly bleak path. But as it turned out, there were others. Some I'd never considered taking, some I'd never imagined taking, and some—most, actually—I'd never imagined whatsoever. But it was that one, wide, scary superhighway

to the worst possible outcome that first held my attention, because it was so… so… so *obvious*. But here's the deal: everything was so *un*real. Any sense of normalcy was gone, including any assumptions about the future. There was absolutely nothing familiar to grab onto. So why should *anything* be obvious? Why would that path to pain and death be any more real than anything else now? So we didn't take that path. It shrunk up and took its place among all the other paths leading off to who knows where. And we started looking around this bizarre Wonderland for anything that might say "Eat Me," or "Drink Me"…

Help wanted

In another lifetime I was sitting on a bench with my buddy, Doug, in a small town in France trying to recover from jetlag and watching several concurrent games of boules played by men (mostly) of all ages in the village square. It was serious business. A guy in the group closest to us was lining up his next toss when a neighborhood mutt without any sense of propriety trotted across the clay and deposited a steaming load directly in the bowler's trajectory. The player straightened up, whistled loudly, and out of nowhere zipped in a young man riding what was essentially a vacuum cleaner the size of a golf cart; he swiftly sucked up the offending pile and then returned to wherever he'd come from, presumably awaiting the next summons. Play resumed without comment. Doug and I looked at each other: "Did you see that? Was that amazing? Who would want that job?"

Well, I'm not sure anyone really wants that job. On the plus side: you get to ride around on a cool little cart in Provence during the summer, making sure others can pursue their activities without interference. On the minus side: you end up every day with a hopper full of dog shit.

Actually, caregiving can be a lot like that—even worse if you don't find a place to dump the hopper full of dog shit. For a position no one really wants to find themself in, the primary caregiver role turned out to be one I had to fight for. Several years earlier I had a blue period, like Picasso, though not as long or productive as his. Then I had a black period. Then I had a black-and-blue period.

I'm not entirely convinced I was clinically depressed since it was largely work-related, but it doesn't make much difference. Ultimately, well before Diana's diagnosis, I traded the anti-depressant for a granddaughter and wrote myself back to life through poetry that has since been confiscated and kept under guard in a Nevada salt mine.

At the time, Diana found this profound change in my outlook perplexing. So did I. If I were questioned under a bare bulb with my feet in water and wires alligator clipped to sensitive places, I'd eventually say I discovered during that time that: 1) I'm not at my most creative during periods of high stress; 2) I want to feel like I'm in control of my own fate; and 3) I'm generally uncomfortable with uncertainty.

In addition, I don't hide my emotions well. Due to our differing childhood circumstances, Diana developed the strength and skills to deal with trauma that I never had to, so she was considerably more stoic, at least outwardly, during the first weeks of diagnosis. I actually felt borderline dehydrated most of that time, but only when the two of us were alone together. The rest of the time I would just curl up and bury my face in a pile of dirty clothes on our closet floor, since lack of privacy was the flip side of being continually supported by friends and family.

I'm not sure Diana thought I was up to the task of taking care of her; it probably looked more like she'd have to take care of me. I wondered about that myself, to a certain extent. And there were plenty of people willing to do the job of primary caregiver. That was one of the factors that led me to step up to it, frankly. I had been hip-checked off the bed in mid-contraction during the birth of our second child because someone in the room thought they were a better coach. I was too stunned at the time to react, so I let it happen. This was a quarter century ago. I hadn't thought about it since, but it popped into my head when I began to receive

so many gracious and generous offers from family and friends to do anything and everything we could ask or need.

But this role was mine. I didn't claim it so much as I reclaimed it. I became proprietary about it. I appreciated all the help—and caregiving does indeed require a lot of help. But the depression I'd felt a couple of years ago had left me with the feeling that I had some making up to do, and now it looked like I might not have enough time to do it.

That said, the caregiving job started getting easier as soon as the final diagnosis was reached. As much as anticipation can often be better than whatever lies ahead, it can also be worse. At least we now knew what we were dealing with, and that made all kinds of choices easier. For instance, the question of how much money we'd need for retirement had seemed to dominate every dinner discussion with friends in the months leading up to the diagnosis. Retirement? What retirement? Retirement had dropped off the radar altogether. So what's the solution to any nagging problem? Easy: Get a bigger one. Here's one place where size does indeed matter.

The Love-In

For Diana's 50th birthday I had whisked her away to a romantic weekend, just the two of us. For my 50th, Diana surprised me with a huge party with friends and family from near and far. I gave her what I wanted in a party, and she gave me what she wanted. So it all worked out. We had nothing scheduled for the weekend that fell between the suspicion that the cancer was really bad and the confirmation that it was even worse. I figured we'd spend it deciding which wall to stare at blankly, or maybe making an effort to string two consecutive thoughts together, when Diana suddenly announced: "Let's have a party!"

If there was anything—*anything* in the world—I wanted to do less, I couldn't come up with it. I was trying to marshal all the reasons why this was a bad idea, but if thoughts were hard to come by, words were even harder. So I trained my blank stare on Diana and said, "Sure."

Whereas my reasoning was nonexistent, Diana's was sound. Sharing news of a recent cancer diagnosis can be depleting, and only a handful of friends knew of her condition. Once word got out, we'd be inundated with calls and concern. Diana was going to perform a preemptive strike and get it over with all at once. We assumed she would be heading into traditional chemo and radiation treatments soon, so while she already didn't feel great, she would only feel worse in the coming weeks.

Diana sent out a blanket email on Thursday announcing the party on Sunday and included a brief summary of what we

knew of her condition. In a moment of inspiration, she called it "The Great South Whidbey Love-In" (South Whidbey is the island near Seattle where we live). And since she knew most of our friends only *pretended* to have been to a love-in, Diana laid out the rules for the party: 1) hug everyone and everything; 2) sing, dance, laugh, and/or engage in scintillating conversation; and 3) under no circumstances discuss anything medical with anyone during the party. She also added that in the spirit of the '60s, hot sex was encouraged, but suggested that anyone so inclined should tie a sock to the doorknob or bush to warn any passersby.

It was an impossible invitation. I mean the whole idea, not just the sex part. I'm pretty sure no one *wanted* to come. *I* didn't want to come. I can only imagine the cajoling, pleading, and threatening that went on among our friends. But at 5:00 p.m. on the day of the party, somewhere in the neighborhood of 125 friends and family dressed in bell bottoms and flower-power garb tripped the light fantastic and showed up at our front door.

Diana figured she could last three hours at most, so she had set an 8:00 p.m. end time for the party. When the last guest left at 11:00 p.m., Diana was in a state of pure bliss. She had been on her feet dancing, singing, and hugging for six hours and she felt better than she did when the party started. And I'm pretty sure everyone who came did, too, but if not, they hid it extremely well. They stuck to her rules. Somewhere between the first beer and the last group hug, the barely detectable pain and sorrow behind our friends' eyes completely disappeared, and Diana was floating above it all like the blessed haze over a Grateful Dead concert.

The effect of the Love-in on Diana was profound—and pivotal. The high carried her through the following week in which each doctor visit provided progressively worse news. Since we were still ten days from a final diagnosis and the beginning of any medical

treatment, Diana views the Love-in as her first chemo infusion. The endorphins coursing through her system were 100% effective in making her feel better; no traditional therapy can come close to that. To whatever treatment protocol the doctors prescribed in the coming weeks, Diana would add her own: she was going to look for Love and Joy *every* day. It is a regimen she has maintained going on eight years. That is Diana's genius.

The idea of throwing a party to announce a diagnosis of cancer would not have occurred to me in a thousand lifetimes. This has nothing to do with experience or education; it's simply a catastrophic failure of the imagination. Mine clearly needed some exercise. As my good friend Dr. Ward Trueblood advised, in reference to a different matter that will remain undisclosed, "Use it or lose it."

Round up

A metastatic cancer is one that, like Wal-Mart, has branched out from its original site and taken up residence elsewhere. In Diana's case, pieces had broken off the mass in her left lung and gone into her lymph nodes, right lung, brain, and possibly into the fluid-that-shouldn't-have-been-there around her heart. From the oncologist's perspective, there is no cure when this happens with lung cancer, and any discussion of "getting rid of it" becomes moot. The idea is that it's too late: if we know the cancer has gone *some*where, it could be *any*where. Instead of a localized cancer, it has become systemic. The cat's out of the bag. The train has left the station. The horses are out of the barn.

Have these guys never seen a '50s Hollywood Western? The horses *always* get out of the barn and the ranchers *always* round 'em up—and often come back with wild horses to boot. How hard can it be?

Pretty damned difficult, according to the medical community. In its view, the only way Diana won't die of lung cancer is if she dies of something else first, like getting hit by a bus. So while our oncologist said he couldn't offer anything that would make Diana better, he was determined to not do anything to make her worse. For that, we are eternally grateful. He prescribed Tarceva, a nontraditional chemotherapy in the form of a daily pill that might—at best—slow the cancer some. It had the benefit of minimal, manageable side effects. He also recommended a highly targeted radiation for the lesions in her brain, a treatment that can be repeated if necessary.

Lung cancer is fast, but brain cancer is faster.

On the morning of the gamma knife treatment for Diana's brain lesions, the radiologist could only find two to treat, whereas the week before there had been three. One of the horses had made its way back to the barn by itself. I asked the radiologist where the third lesion went as he blew though the waiting room. I understood him to say maybe they misread the first MRI. Diana asked him the same question in the treatment room, and she heard, "Who knows? But it's not there now!" So they zapped the two remaining lesions and we went home.

One of the keys to a happy marriage is following Diana's practice of focusing on the qualities one appreciates in one's spouse and overlooking the irritations. I am unbelievably lucky that she figures that I have no more than a 3% annoyance component, a number with which I am completely happy. Part of that 3%, however, is the occasional "correction" that I interject into a story she's telling, such as "Monday. It was on a Monday, not a Tuesday." In my defense, it's not an uncommon habit. It's a niche; somebody has to fill it.

When I hear Diana excitedly tell someone on the phone that perhaps she had meditated the third lesion away, I try to clarify that it might not have been there in the first place. She is stunned—and undone. "How can you not support me?" she asks, in tears. Now I am stunned—and undone.

I come from a reductionist and literal tradition, Diana from a more synthesizing and imaginative one. I am from the sciences; Diana from the humanities. This isn't to say we aren't fairly adept at wandering in the other's field, but in a time of crisis it's easier to fall back on the familiar. When my head wasn't spinning out of control during this diagnosis and early treatment period, I was frantically trying to make some sense of things from a clinical, biological point of view. Diana was already moving toward a narrative,

the development of a personal mythology that could chart a way through this. (This is not myth as in "made-up story," but as in Joseph Campbell's definition of an epic heroic journey—the travails and triumphs of a life lived, not the tragedy of a life ending.) Given this disparity in our personal foundations, the difference between a lesion being "not ever there" and "there, but now gone" was fantastically huge, and completely unappreciated by me at the time.

We learned two things from this episode: 1) make sure we're both in the room whenever we talk to the doctors so we're both hearing the same thing, and 2) we're going to need help with our communications if we're going to get through this.

Whose life is it, anyway?

And now we get to the part of the story where I feel sorry for myself.

My aversion to psychotherapy wasn't based on personal experience, because I had no personal experience of therapy. That's because I had an aversion to it. If there's a good reason for that, it's buried somewhere deep and I'd need help digging it up. That's not going to happen.

I did not, however, have an aversion to therapists, because some of my friends were therapists. I had no way of knowing if they were any good, though. The only therapist that I knew for sure was any good was Sarri Gilman, who practiced in the nearby town of Langley—and she was much better than good. Sarri helped Diana through the residual effects of a difficult adolescent trauma that had oozed for decades before eventually becoming an open sore that needed attention. Sarri helped Diana immeasurably. And I trusted her unequivocally—and still do. That doesn't mean I wanted to see her, though.

However, after our uncharacteristic meltdown about the reason behind the mysterious missing lesion—and, yes, on Diana's insistence—I was willing to go with her to see Sarri. I was still reeling from the pain of the diagnosis and the shock of Diana's accusation that I wasn't supporting her, and I was expecting something along the lines of making sure we communicated clearly and often.

But instead what I heard was that this was Diana's story, first and foremost, and that it was held together by the thinnest thread of hope. Anything that might compromise that would be detrimental to Diana's fragile health. I didn't disagree, but I was surprised that I would have to keep to myself any misgiving, misunderstanding, or even simple request for clarification I might have.

I looked to Diana to see if she agreed with Sarri, and her brief nod was enough to let me know that access to my sole and trusted confidante of 32 years had vanished, at least for the time being.

"But what if she's wrong?" I asked Sarri.

"Under these circumstances, 'wrong' doesn't play a role," Sarri replied. "Everyone else's story may be right, but Diana's is the only one that matters."

Diana and I had walked into Sarri's office like we were coming off a battlefield: shell-shocked and wounded. Like a good triage doc in a M.A.S.H. unit, Sarri quickly—and accurately—determined that while I was metaphorically covered in blood, it was all Diana's. I would survive; Diana might not. Diana clearly had the stronger need, and the treatment for that was for her to be in complete control of how her life would play out.

This actually made a lot of sense to me. There was just one niggling implication.

"Sooooo… where does this leave me, then?" I asked.

"I'd be happy to work with you separately or refer you to another therapist," Sarri offered. "Or you can look to someone else for support—just not Diana."

But Diana *was* my support. And talking to someone else was problematic. A therapist, even Sarri? Thank you, no. I didn't have a pastor. Or a bartender. And everyone else—family, friends, acquaintances, even people we didn't know well—had all been enlisted in Diana's spiritual army. I felt like I had just been bucked

from co-captain to grunt, and that talking to anyone about any misgivings would be dissension in the ranks. So not wanting to run the risk of doing anything that might be treasonous, I just hunkered down in my foxhole, ankle deep in muck, and sent myself coded messages, which frequently turned out to be beyond my ability to decipher.

Somebody—*anybody*—could have deciphered those messages: "Get out of the damned foxhole!" But it's hard to break a code when it's based on self-pity. There are hundreds of caregiver support groups available, but it didn't occur to me to try one. Besides, they weren't really my style, just like therapy wasn't my style. Neither was journal writing, or talking to anybody else. Stoicism *was* my style. Problem is, my style sort of sucked.

Luckily, Diana's narrative started looking really good, so as soon as I could I jumped on board with it. That's not to say something didn't come up occasionally that I would've liked to question further, but I kept those thoughts to myself. And when anyone would ask how I was, *really*, I'd reply that all things considered, I was doing quite well. And most of the time that would be true.

For Emily, Wherever I May Find Her

—Simon & Garfunkel

The only thing worse for a biology major than thinking the cat in the dissection tray looked familiar was sharing the lab with future doctors. In the eyes of a natural scientist, the sole contribution of premed students to undergraduate education was the ability to horribly skew an otherwise perfectly good grading curve. Thirty-five years later, I'm more appreciative of the doctors and researchers my lab mates became, and I feel honored to have been in a position to further their advancement so early in their careers.

I like doctors. I like nurses. I like hospitals. I like the time I've spent in hospitals. I like knowing where the blanket warmer is, and the vending machines. I like the recliners that let me sleep next to Diana's bed. I like the cafeteria. There have been times when a square of green Jell-O capped by a dollop of something synthetic has rivaled any dessert I've ever had. I like the medical profession and its institutions because they have collectively worked extremely hard to save Diana's life. Of course, I haven't

been sliced, stitched, kneaded, basted, and in unimaginable pain, so it's understandable that, while grateful, Diana has a different association with the experience.

This is just to say that I had no reason to doubt either Diana's diagnosis or prognosis, as bleak and shocking as they were. I had the utmost faith in the sciences in general and the medical community in particular, so hoping the tests were wrong, or that there might be another way through this, didn't occur to me at the time. Before the diagnosis Diana and I had shared a vision of a future, indistinct as it was, that included both of us getting old together. And now that clearly wasn't going to happen. She was going to die. And I was going to keep on living. Without her.

That was hard to get used to.

But getting used to it was vital, otherwise I was going to remain rooted in that realm of disbelief, and therefore be of no use to anyone, especially Diana. I was so distraught by what I was about to lose that I was overlooking what I still had. Two of our coworkers—both with marriages as equally devoted as ours—had abruptly lost their husbands not six months before Diana's diagnosis. Both widows were bravely, but not easily, making their way forward. Life does indeed go on. That put the question of "How can I possibly live without Diana" in perspective. Ironically, letting go of our future—letting go of *Diana*—was what allowed me to focus on her, to appreciate her. I think it's likely that almost any curse in life is followed by a blessing, and this was a blessing for me. Sometimes it's the other way around: the blessing first, then the curse. Sometimes it's hard to know which is which, and only time will tell.

In Thornton Wilder's play, *Our Town*, the newly deceased Emily is sitting in the hillside cemetery with other former inhabitants of Grover's Corners, all of whom are gazing wistfully down at the still-very-much-alive town. Emily bemoans not paying more

attention to the little things in life, regretting how the tedious took precedence over the mundane, when the mundane itself can actually be a marvel. Diana and I started referring to times like these as "Emily moments." They were characterized by having no relation to the ordinary flow of time, having no demands or expectations, just unplanned happenings that ranged from unimpressive ordinariness to unbelievable spectacle. Standing at a rail watching tugboats with my parents on a Sunday afternoon. Seeing the tranquility of a Zen garden in a plowed vacant lot in California's Central Valley. Recognizing Mt. Rainier's shadow on the sky at sunrise before anyone else was up and about. Feeling the trickling warmth across my chest from a sleeping grandchild with an already-saturated Fuzzy Bun. Timeless, magical events whose spell would be broken if we even just *thought* about wishing they would never end.

I figured we had been averaging about five "Emily Days" per year over the past ten years or so; five days that were memorable, distinguishable, and fully appreciated, versus 360 that somehow just melted into each other. At that rate, assuming we had another 30 years or so to live we could look forward to about 150 more Emily Days. The prognosis for Diana was somewhere between a handful of months to a year left to live, which might be about 150 days. So they all had to be Emily Days.

Helplessly Hoping

"… her harlequin hovers nearby…" I love Crosby, Stills & Nash. I love their harmonies, melodies, Martin guitars, and especially their album covers. But their lyrics were always beyond me, so I paid very little attention to them. I get the "helplessly hoping" part, though.

I wasn't alone in this; everyone around us felt helpless. Empathy needs an outlet, and in the absence of anything to *do* our friends and families frequently had something to *give*: books, music, poems, smoothie recipes, cure-all diets, meditation tapes, Native American amulets, Sedona healing crystals, figurines from every cultural tradition, energy bracelets, juju bags, magic talismans, and copies of scriptures in the actual handwriting of Buddha, Mohammed, God, and Dr. Andrew Weil. We appreciated all of it, had no idea what to do with half of it, but still tried most of it even though any given object's inherent powers were quite often extremely well hidden.

Diana incorporated quite a few of these gifts into her daily routine of seeking joy and happiness, and she began to feel… better! I doubted she actually *was* better, but just feeling better was a huge improvement. But there was one particular suggestion offered by our friend April that also made *me*—and anyone else who tried it with Diana—feel better immediately for the sole reason that it was *something to do*.

April is a talented practitioner of a Japanese healing touch method called Jin Shin Jyutsu, something I'd paid absolutely no attention to whatsoever. While April couldn't make it to the Love-in

she had emailed a "mini-treatment" for Diana that anyone in attendance could try if they were either a) so inclined, or b) slightly inebriated. Luckily we were blessed with plenty of both.

I suspect the real name of the treatment probably includes the words "energy" and "harmonizing" or "balance" but it's now known all over the south end of Whidbey Island and throughout our families as "Fingers & Toes." Like most Asian healing touch systems, Jin Shin Jyutsu is based on the idea of energy coursing through the body via meridians, much the way the circulatory system carries blood and the lymphatic system transports lymph. Since most of these energy meridians begin or end in the hands and feet, the Fingers & Toes treatment is focused there. Well, sure, why not?

To administer a treatment, I (or anyone) would sit next to Diana and gently hold the pinky of her left hand in one hand, and the big toe of her right foot in the other. After 20 seconds or so, I'd feel separate pulses in the toe and finger that would usually be out of whack, so I'd wait for them to synch up. That in itself was a little bizarre. Then I'd move to the next finger and toe pair, ending up with the thumb and pinky toe. To close the session with that hand and foot, I'd press the palm of her hand and the sole of her foot and wait for those pulses to synch up. Then I'd move to her other hand and foot and start over. A treatment would typically last anywhere from 5 to 20 minutes.

At first everyone treated this as a parlor game, just something to do, a few moments of sanctioned intimacy with Diana that would otherwise have been socially awkward. Usually, the first treatment someone gave Diana began with what-the-hell nervous laughter, but more often than not ended in a deeper, softer conversation oblivious to the surrounding chaos. Subsequent treatments by the same person frequently yielded no conversation at all, and took on an almost meditative quality.

To be honest, I was just glad there was something for people to do when spending time with Diana, and I didn't pay that much attention to what was happening during a treatment, even when I was the one giving it. Then our sister-in-law Susan observed that Diana's incessant coughing stopped whenever someone gave her a treatment. *That* got my attention. Any time she coughed from that moment on, regardless of where we were, the nearest person reached for Diana's fingers and toes.

The radiologist who performed the procedure on Diana's brain had warned us that more lesions would likely show up in the next MRI. Our oncologist's only hope for the targeted chemo was that it might slow the rate of cancer growth—*if* we were lucky. At Diana's first check-up four weeks after starting on Tarceva and three weeks post-Gamma Knife surgery, her brain MRI showed no new lesions. The CT of her chest showed the main mass in her lung had shrunk by half. Something was happening in Diana's body that couldn't be credited exclusively to her medical care.

That *really* got my attention.

The Mending Wall

Something there is that doesn't love a wall
And wants it down...

—Robert Frost

Not only was my mind *not* a fertile field for anything that smacked of New Age, but it was surrounded by a wall topped with razor wire and broken glass. There's a fine line between skepticism and cynicism and I'm sure I've stumbled across it a time or two, but I don't think of myself as a cynic. And I'm not entirely convinced that I'm even skeptical by nature, but training and experience have led me to examine anything beyond the ordinary with, let's say, suspicion.

I believe in the scientific process and I have a mechanical mind that hums along to a walking bass line of cause and effect. A sound hypothesis speaks to me; a nuanced theory can be positively seductive; but each has to have some substance, some credibility, some basis other than just wishing it were so. I have found the simplicities and contortions of religion restrictive, conspiracies tedious, and alternate realities arbitrary. I have wielded Occam's Razor like a Cuisinart, slicing and dicing suspect arguments into bits and pieces that wilt under the glare of mathematical probability.

At least, that has been my reputation. And as reputations are prone to do, it had broken free of its chains and chased any make and model of idea that went down our street, leaving me standing

on the porch in horror, half wishing it'd get hit. It's easy to get a reputation; it's much harder to train it.

Somewhere along the line, I stopped applying intellectual rigor to extraordinary events or concepts I would read or hear about and just automatically jump to the conclusion that I had reached so often before: Bah, humbug. I found myself short-circuiting the very scientific process I accused others of hijacking. Nowhere was this more evident than when our friend April told us about the finger/toes Jin Shin treatment. But as soon as we realized that Diana stopped coughing during the treatment... bah, hmmmmmm....

Keep doing what you're doing and you'll keep getting what you're getting. That's not from ancient Greece; it's from a Chinese fortune cookie. I was already painfully familiar with its corollary during high school: Keep doing what you're doing and you'll keep not getting what you're not getting. Anything we were doing or not doing that held even the remotest possibility of stopping Diana's cough was worth investigating, but it still surprised me as much as anybody that I climbed onto the Jin Shin Jyutsu life raft when our ship sank. Why I would do this was not nearly as interesting—or as perplexing—to me as how this raft could possibly float?

I'm pretty sure it has something to do with physics. As far as I can tell, there are energy sinks and then there are energy *synchs*, and you don't need to be a rocket scientist to know the difference. The first is easy: energy, like water, seeks the lowest possible level, typically the sofa. The second is more complicated, and involves independent energy sources seeking each other and inexplicably establishing a corresponding rhythmicity.

Diana and I avoided energy sinks, whether they were people, situations, or states of mind. But we actively sought energy synchs, with Jin Shin being our introduction to the concept. Holding Diana's fingers and toes was initially just an exercise in weirdness,

and I'd typically just hold each pair for a while and move on to the next, with my mind wandering off as I did so. After a few treatments, though, I started to feel the pulses immediately, without the twenty or thirty-second delay. Some days they would be wildly out of whack and would take a while to synchronize; other days they were aligned from the start.

So what are these pulses? Energy meridians? Cardiac pulses? Emanations from the rings of Saturn? Are they really two independent internal pulses in Diana's body? Or in mine? Or one in each? The question seemed important to me, so I delved into the literature about acupressure, acupuncture, chakras, Ayurvedic medicine, and healing touch methods of all kinds.

April sent us more treatments to try, as well as an introductory Jin Shin book. I devoured it. I made flash cards of the points and meridians and carried them around with me. Later I drew the meridians on a Ken doll so I could see them all at a glance, and study their relationships. (*"Pops, why do you have a naked doll with no hair and colored lines on it?" "All grandfathers have these, Thea. Papa Steve probably has one, too."*) Jin Shin is essentially a Japanese subset of Chinese acupressure, but with only 26 points. Instead of pinpoint precision, just getting within a couple of inches is close enough to be effective.

I'm sure purists would scream at this, but all of the energy systems seem to me to be fundamentally the same, so I let myself be guided by Diana's standard of "Does this make it better or worse?" After early treatments in which I was often preoccupied with a sequence of points, counting how long to hold, or pondering "Cloud Gate," "Lesser Rushing," "Nonfat Nofoam," and the names of other points, I eventually settled into balancing sequences and then let my hands roam—not too far, usually—to where they felt drawn. I know, it sounds bizarre. Oh, and I also light candles.

I never came across a really satisfactory answer about the pulses, but before long I didn't need one. I could feel *something*, and it didn't matter to me what it was. Diana could feel it, too. When I put my hands directly over the mass in her lung, it would feel like her entire chest was a bubbling cauldron under my palms. After a few minutes, the chaotic syncopations would resolve into a steady, slow, single pulse. I don't know what that's about. And I don't care. The treatments were good for both of us.

The Standards

*S*tardust. *Take the "A" Train. Round Midnight.* Any jazz musician worth his chops knows these tunes and others like them, collectively known in the trade as "The Standards." They are all recognizable and popular with the general audience. When all else fails, resort to a Standard. The smiles will get bigger and so will the tips.

Think Positive. Be Optimistic. Have a Good Attitude. These are also Standards, the fallback positions of a well-wisher in full retreat from knowing what else to say. If I had a buck for each time I heard (or said myself) something along those lines, we wouldn't have needed health insurance. *It Don't Mean a Thing (If It Ain't Got That Swing).*

It's not that it's bad advice; I just didn't find it very helpful. The first problem I see is that each of these qualities—positive, optimistic, good—is a relative measure, but it sounds like it's supposed to be an absolute, some kind of immutable safe haven without any clear consensus on how to get there. The second problem is the inherent assumption that there's a conscious choice involved, and sometimes there is, but quite often there isn't. The third problem I have with it is it says one thing but means another. It's not necessarily an invitation to go somewhere, but a lightly sweetened admonition *not* to go somewhere else: Don't get stuck in the muck.

Now *that's* actually good advice. Getting down in the muck is unavoidable, and maybe even wallowing in it a bit, but getting

stuck there is decidedly unhelpful. Advising someone to be happy, though, is not the same thing as encouraging them *not* to be sad. There is a considerable amount of neutral ground between the two.

I felt no compulsion to work myself into an unsupportable optimistic lather, but there were several things that I found helpful in hosing off the muck after Diana's diagnosis. I think of these as my own personal Standards, but since I also think they can help anyone in dire straits—and because this is just the way my mind works—I'm going to express them as universal theorems, without apology.

There are apparently lots of variations on the **existence theorem,** most involving mathematical abstractions, philosophical caveats, and a smattering of Latin expressions. They're of no practical use whatsoever. But my friend Jim Stanley once netted it out like this: It's easier to do something if you know it's been done before.

When Diana was diagnosed, our niece Jesse told us that the mother of a friend of a friend had been diagnosed with Stage IV lung cancer and went into remission. That was enough to open the door to possibility. In retrospect, we didn't know anything at all about the woman, her circumstances, her treatment, or her outlook. Even now we don't know her current situation—or even if the report of her remission was accurate. Or if she existed at all, for that matter. So I'll modify the existence theorem: It's easier to do something if you know, suspect, or even mistakenly believe it has been done before.

That brings us to the **inevitability theorem.** Just because there's no scientific or anecdotal evidence of something being done before doesn't mean it can't happen. There was a first man to walk on the moon. A first black woman to sit in the front of the bus. Wile E. Coyote will eventually catch The Roadrunner. There's always a first time, no matter what the odds. The latest cosmological theories

support the idea of a limitless multiverse consisting of an infinite number of universes, and we live in one of them. (Or rather I live in one; you may live in another.) If that's the case, then the discussion of odds becomes moot. The chance of one in anything doesn't just mean it *can* happen, but that it *will* happen. Perhaps you're in the universe where it does. Diana and I were.

And the last one is the **miracle/schmiracle theorem.** Depending on who you ask, miracles are either hard to come by or a dime a dozen; disbursed at the discretion of the divine according to some, or apparent in every waking moment according to others. Was it a miracle that the third lesion in Diana's brain disappeared before treatment? Yes, no, maybe so. What difference does it make? If you don't believe in miracles but suddenly find yourself in the market for one, remember that an unexplained mystery is just as good—and they're everywhere.

Please don't misunderstand. I'm not disparaging optimism. I think it's wonderful. If there's anything at all to the notion of self-fulfilling prophecies, it makes sense to hold a vision of the future that works out rather than one that doesn't. But I don't see that as optimism, it's just common sense—and even that is sometimes difficult to maintain when all evidence appears to be to the contrary, no matter what someone advises you. That's when I found the theorems to come in handy.

Chin up. *Take Five.*

Deviant behavior

Cozying up by the fire with a good book. Cuddling on the couch with a kitty. Huddling on the hearth with a mug of hot chocolate. Snuggling on the sofa with a soft statistic. You don't hear that last one much. That's because statistics aren't warm and fuzzy, even the good ones. The bad ones are downright mean. And none of them are personal.

I didn't search the web for information about Diana's condition or prospects. I was pretty sure what I'd find. Diana, on the other hand, *did* search, and she found exactly what I was afraid she would. Nothing good, and everything bad. Very bad. The lung cancer sites—at least in 2006—were bleaker than bleak, lacking anything to counter or offset the prognosis offered by the medical community. Diana shut down her computer. I just shut down.

As useful as statistics are in evaluating *probabilities* in large populations, they are completely worthless in determining *possibility* in individuals. Diana somehow intuited that distinction; had it occurred to me, I would have discounted it. I believed in numbers, even when they told me something that made me absolutely sick. Numbers don't lie.

But they don't tell the whole truth, either. So we were lucky that our oncologist emphasized that any published clinical study is based on data from what *has* happened, using protocols that existed *then*, and a sample population that—and this is most important—*did not include Diana*. That's a considerable margin of error for whatever was going to happen next.

That also got me thinking about the standard deviation. This is the metric in any study that accounts for the variation of the test subjects. A low number means the responses of the subjects were similar; a high number means the responses were all over the map. The standard deviation is an average, so even a low number could include a subject that was wildly different from all the rest. Since the outlook presented by the studies for lung cancer was dismal, the message was clear: be deviant. Get crazy. Go wild. Do *not* be normal. Diana got to this idea early and on her own; I didn't even have to bring up the standard deviation.

With so much unfiltered, unexplained, and unverified information just a website away, it's easy to be sucked in by statistics. My advice to anyone in a seemingly hopeless situation is this: stay off the cancer sites, or any other site that addresses what ails you. And have garlic or holy water handy just in case a nightmare statistic suddenly materializes out of nowhere.

Bad boys and girls

Diana's cancer wasn't an interloper, an invader, or an infection. This cancer didn't come from a virus or bacteria, though some cancers apparently do. This hodge-podge of a mass in her left lung, the outliers in her right, the bloated lymph nodes, the lesions in her brain, the wayfaring cells plying the pericardial effusion were all Diana's very own cells, as much a part of her as any of her other cells. Wayward cells, maybe, but still hers.

These were the bad boys hanging out in the parking lot, cutting class, and smoking. These were the girls-gone-wild on Spring Break, stripping off the civility of local custom and showing just how bad they could be. These were anarchists, nonconformists, bohemian artists who weren't out to paint a pretty picture; the anti-establishment hippies doin' their own thing, rippin' off The Man, hangin' in the Haight—free-love types that were indiscriminately multiplying and seemingly convincing others to join them.

But since many of my closest and dearest friends belonged to one or more of those groups at one time, I found it a little difficult to come down real hard on Diana's cancer cells. So I decided that I'd spend my time during the Jin Shin Fingers & Toes treatments having a conversation with them, instead of visualizing death rays from my fingertips blasting them all to oblivion.

From the very beginning, during a Jin Shin treatment, Diana could access a visual vocabulary and inference in her meditations that Fellini couldn't have imagined and Freud could only dream of. This has served her extremely well. I, on the other hand, had to

take my cues from Dale Carnegie's *How to Win Friends & Influence People* and the hostage negotiators on TV cop shows.

Okay, tumor cells here's the deal: you're a fun bunch obviously having a good time, but look down the road a bit. This can't last. You're generally making a nuisance of yourselves, and you've started stealing from the neighbors. They're upset, and they're calling the cops. If you keep drawing this much attention to yourselves, you're going to get hit, hard. Radiation. Toxic chemicals. Surgery. This won't be a happy place anymore. You have to go, and I don't mean go somewhere else; I mean go as in 'go away'. First stop doing what you're doing, and then just stop being what you're being. Turn yourselves in. Donate yourselves to science. Let the macrophages, t-cells, and leucocytes help clean up the mess you're making and recycle your parts. Some of you guys are seriously whacked, so take yourselves all the way down to amino acids and nucleotides. You'll feel better for it. 'Tis a far, far better thing....'

You get the idea.

I started having this one-sided conversation with Diana's cancer every time we did the Fingers & Toes, so at least once a day. At the end of the first month following her diagnosis, the main mass in her lung had decreased by half. The scans during the following several months showed it had diminished further, and all the other areas had resolved. Now this could've been due to a lot of things, and it's likely that it was some or all of them together. Or—even though it rarely works on TV—it could've been that I talked the bad boys down, just as simple as that.

Tool Time

"Right tool for the right job," my dad always says, and not only does he likely have the specialized tool necessary for an arcane one-off job, but he can reliably put his finger on it when needed. Sadly, that is not an inheritable trait, so I try to emulate MacGyver of '80s TV who could use his Swiss Army Knife and objects at hand, such as dental floss and a condom, to construct a hot air balloon and fly to Nicaragua. My exploits, however, are typically limited to using a bent soda straw to tighten a Phillips-head screw.

The problem we faced in dealing with Diana's lung cancer was not knowing what, exactly, were the right tools? The medical community made it clear to us that it didn't have them. It had some big tools, some good tools, and some brand-new tools—but not enough tools. Everyone else had plenty of suggestions, though, about what to try, what to eat, what to think, what to do, and—since Dealing with Stage IV Hopeless Lung Cancer is a Do-It-Yourself project without a recommended tool list—we tried them all. Well, not them all. We reviewed anything ingestible with our oncologist who scratched a few off the list as possibly interfering with the molecular mechanism driven by Tarceva (Diana's daily chemo pill), and he looked on the rest as "well, they're not going to hurt" more than "they might very well help."

But something very well *did* help. The CTs and MRIs that first summer continued to show remarkable results that couldn't be explained by Tarceva alone. So what was it? Vitamin D? Jin Shin? Smoothies? Visualizations? Meditations? Massage? Walks? Talks?

The fungus that grows on the backs of caterpillars in the misty mountains traversed by the Great Wall of China? Since we didn't know which were the right tools, we kept using them all and, in fact, kept adding to them. But if I were stranded on a desert island with a Stage IV Lung Cancer patient and had to choose just one tool to have with me… I'd choose our granddaughter, Thea.

I don't know why the idea of time travel and time machines is such a big deal in literature, movies, and imaginations. Traveling forward or backward in time is easy. I used to spend at least half my time preoccupied about the future and the other half recollecting—okay, reinventing—the past. It's the here-and-now that's been most elusive for me. That's what I'd like to have had a machine or a tool for, to anchor me in whatever moment I happened to be in, neither overwhelmed by where Diana's cancer came from nor incapacitated by where it could go.

That's what I think Thea did for us. She was just 9 months old when Diana was diagnosed, so she was inalterably fixed in the present, unconcerned and unaffected by recent events and the possibility of her grandmother's truncated future. In the midst of the tumult and uncertainty of those first months, she was the natural light sunlamp so many of us rely on in the Northwest, the transdermal patch that provided whatever prescriptive remedy we needed, the tether that kept us from going anywhere, forward or back.

My favorite line from *Citizen Kane* is "Yesterday is history, tomorrow's a mystery, today is a gift. That's why it's called 'the present.'" Okay, it's actually from *Kung Fu Panda*, and there's nothing original about it. But it runs continuously in a special venue of my heart because that was the movie playing for Thea's first trip to the Blue Fox Drive-In movie theater in Oak Harbor, which she absolutely loved. Plus we've watched it on DVD about 500 times since. That has also kept me from going anywhere.

Traps

As an engineering marvel, the P-trap of a typical bathroom sink ranks right up there with shadow puppetry and Frank Gehry's Experience Music Project in Seattle—and is equally unappreciated. The P-trap is that deep bend in the plumbing between the drain and the wall beneath any bathroom sink. The water retained in the P-trap prevents the sewer gas on the downstream side of the trap from sneaking back into a house. The P-trap is what allowed the outhouse to come in from the cold.

I was a P-trap for Diana, shielding her from the rare but toxic back flush from the occasional misguided well-wisher, and from anything else she shouldn't have to deal with, such as garden-variety reality. And I was the outlet for Diana's own exceedingly rare but bleak episodes that were better sent down the drain at night than aired in the light of day. That was my job. I was pretty good at it. But as with any case of standing water, which is fundamental to the design of a good P-trap, things settle out. And accumulate.

That was my problem too, so next-door nephew John and son-in-law Isaac took it upon themselves to take me out every once in a while for a good cleaning on the golf course. I wasn't sure that was what I needed, to be honest, since golf can be more infuriating than relaxing, but I figured they were desperate for some way to help out, so I decided to help them by letting them help me. That kind of convoluted thinking exactly mirrored the way I played.

The golf I had learned was a rather genteel sport, in which a nice easy swing was supposedly preferable to something with

more... oomph. More Barry Manilow than Smashing Pumpkins. But after yet another safe and somewhat distracted swing that sent my ball careening into someone's yard anyway, Isaac solemnly suggested, "Why don't you just hit it as hard as you'd really like to?" "Yeah," John agreed, "if you're going to get a penalty stroke, at least earn it."

Those two comments made all the difference for me. They actually hurt my score considerably, but helped my psyche immeasurably. They cleared up any question about who was helping whom. John and Isaac both flirted with low handicaps the more we played, while I was just under par for any given round—if we only counted my penalty strokes. But let's face it: score keeping can be rather arbitrary. Sometimes accepted measures and indications—whether on a scorecard, blood test, or multimillion-dollar medical machinery—don't accurately reflect the best part of a story. Sometimes you just have to count something else.

A formerly well-respected professional golfer who shall remain nameless (yep, that's the guy) once referred to golf as a game of recovery. No matter what horrible lie we might have, the next shot could get us out of it. Whether I found myself in the sand trap, the P-trap, or even the trap of complacency, it was good to keep in mind that whatever happened next could change everything, as could whatever happened right after that. What *isn't* a game of recovery?

Prince of Darkness

I am a product of the age of the atom, when the fun and folly of duck-and-cover drills first revealed to me if not a chink in the armor of my much-adored 3rd-grade teacher, then at least rust on the rivets. Crouching on my hands and knees, forehead pressed against the cool linoleum floor, I knew my desk wasn't going to protect me from an atomic bomb. It couldn't even protect me from Buddy Brittain.

In addition to holding the world hostage with the threat of imminent annihilation, the Atomic Age also captured the American imagination through the cheesy horrors of low-budget movies of the '50s. I saw my first film, *Creature from the Black Lagoon,* as a toddler at the Big Lake Drive-in in West Texas. My parents had assumed I'd be asleep by the time they drove the 48 miles to get to the theater. They were wrong. Nor did I sleep for the next fifteen years. Or go swimming. But I *was* hooked.

I'm pretty sure I've seen every B-grade creature feature Hollywood ever produced. So I should've been completely prepared for the possibility that some amorphous radioactive blob of toxic chemicals could appear without warning, lay waste to the neighborhood, and threaten to devour the future-as-we-expect-it along with a handful of hapless bikini-clad teenagers. That sounds an awfully lot like the diagnosis of late-stage cancer. It sounds even more like the conventional *treatment* for late-stage cancer.

We were lucky that Diana was able to avoid conventional treatments. That in itself eliminated most of the monsters. But not

all of them. This *is* a horror movie, after all. Even now it's hard to know in real life where I am in the movie. The triumphant ending? Or the triumphant *false* ending with another 20 minutes to go?

In movies, the malevolence you don't see is so much worse than the one you do. As a horror-movie buff, I find the phantasm more terrifying than the fantastic. The less screen time something gets, the more incapacitating it is when it appears. As a caregiver, I found it worked the same way. The certainty of the diagnosis, the visual evidence of the scans, even the dismal prospects for Diana's survival somehow became less frightening as they became more apparent. Knowing what the monster looked like and how it was likely to behave was half the battle. The other half was the anticipation of how it would all play out: the fear, pain, sadness, anger, and uncertainty.

Caregivers often refer to this part as a "darkness." That's a pretty apt description for something that comes and goes at will, and obscures all else even at a time when things appear to be going quite well given the circumstances.

Once past the first month or so from diagnosis, this shadowy netherworld descended upon me very rarely, probably less than one percent of the time. But when it did, there was nothing one-percent about it; it was a 100% all-consuming pitch black.

Darkest just before the dawn. Light dispels darkness. Light at the end of the tunnel. Every dark cloud has a silver lining. There, that's out of the way. I might've found those helpful *outside* the darkness, but never from within it.

For me, anger didn't play a big role. That Diana, a non-smoker, would get lung cancer was shocking, not unjust. It was unjust even for *smokers* to get lung cancer. That she would be leaving me alone wasn't her fault, or the fault of anyone else. And once I learned of the arsenal of narcotics and anesthetics available to her should she

need them, the anticipated pain of standing by while Diana suffered pretty much dispersed. My own blend of susceptibilities that fed the darkness was made up of 43% fear, 31% uncertainty, and 97% sadness. Don't even try to make those add up right. That's just how it works. Even worse, these were overlaid by the self-recrimination that I shouldn't let myself feel any of them.

That, of course, is utter nonsense. I'm a Darwinist at heart, so if something exists then it likely confers some kind of evolutionary advantage, metaphorically if not actually. This darkness serves a purpose. So what is it? I'd guess it's different for everyone, but I experienced it in several ways:

1. As **before-the-fact mourning** for Diana's imminent death, sadness over the loss of our future together, and a nostalgic review of our lives to-date that magically enhanced already-fond recollections and repaved any rough patches;

2. As a **hedge against pie-in-the-sky delusion**, a reminder that the situation remained serious and the cancer likely had its own agenda;

3. And—as hard as it may be to believe and as much as I hate to admit it—as an **escape**… a personal, private, and safe place to retreat from *everything*. In retrospect, it was probably my introduction to the concept of "being completely present," of pure unadulterated being-ness. The darkness could be, ironically, a very comforting and seductive place. I could consider any gloomy possibility that occurred to me without burdening Diana (*especially* Diana) or anyone else with it, and without the worry that it would somehow manifest itself. (Scary movie rule #43: *Never* read the Latin inscription aloud.)

So if darkness has a purpose, that means it is essentially a tool and therefore has a limited useful life. Once it has either worn out or accomplished its goal, it will no longer be needed. Once Tokyo was destroyed, Godzilla returned to the sea. Once the zombie eats your brain, he leaves you alone.

The passage of time helped, but I also wanted to stop feeding the demon. I got over the pre-mourning fairly quickly as it seemed I had a very limited time left with Diana, and I didn't want to waste it. I wasn't in any danger of overlooking the seriousness of our situation, so I didn't think I really needed the hedge against delusion after a while. In fact, I was thinking delusion was considerably more helpful than the hedge by that time. So that was two down.

Getting rid of the safe haven aspect was a bit more complicated. I had felt a distinct *need* to first avoid and then later confront all the ugly possibilities ahead of me and, yes, to feel sorry for myself. I think that's natural. I was *entitled* to spend time in the darkness. I *deserved* it, right? Well... noooo, not really. A certain amount of self-preservation in these circumstances serves a higher master; self-indulgence does not. As the needle swung more toward the latter, it was time to get rid of whatever the beast was after.

Darkness is the absence of imagination, not illumination. I haven't had a walking dead, wraith, radioactive lizard, or anything else hiding in my closet for quite some time. All it took to dispel the last vestige of darkness was to think the unthinkable, to consider something I would've recoiled from had someone mentioned it to me when Diana was first diagnosed. But as soon as I entertained the possibility that a future could theoretically exist in which the best possible outcome for *both* of us could be that Diana *does not survive*—and that I could be okay with that—the darkness disappeared.

So yes, I drove a stake through my own heart. That's not just a monster. It's a bitch.

Misfortune telling

Diagnosis, prognosis, ceanothus. The last is a flowering shrub that left untended overwhelmed our entire flowerbed. The second threatened to do the same thing to my psyche. The first comes from the Greek roots "dia" (through, between, across, apart) and "gnosis" (to know). With the medical imaging currently available, to know through/between/across/apart is pretty accurate; a misdiagnosis is much more rare than it used to be. Prognosis is a different story. "Pro" means "before, forward, in place of." Before knowing. Knowing the future. In place of knowing. This is crystal ball stuff. To be sure, prognoses are based on a wealth of experience, but misprognoses are fairly common. If they are any more accurate than stock market predictions, it's only because the monkeys throwing darts are wearing lab coats. In this era of consumer protection and truth in advertising, I propose we call prognoses what they really are: Proguesses.

The professional prognosis for Diana of 3 to 12 months to live nearly killed me and I wasn't even the patient. Diana accepted the diagnosis, and if she didn't outright reject the prognosis, she at least ignored it. I think that pissed it off and it took it out on me. It didn't occur to me that the prognosis could be wrong until we were past the one-year mark, the outside date of her expected demise, and even then I only allowed (to myself) that it was maybe "sorta wrong."

Now we're eight years out and Diana is for all intents and purposes completely healthy. From the western medical perspective it's as close as she'll get to being cured in the realm of Stage IV

cancer. So doesn't that make the initial prognosis wrong? Well, no. It's not that the prognosis was wrong exactly, it's just that it wasn't exactly right, either.

I painted houses one summer to earn money for college. By the end of July I had developed an aversion to shingled siding and an appreciation for subjective statistics. My partner, Harry, figured we had a 50/50 chance of getting a job at each door we knocked on because the house either needed painting or it didn't. I suggested that by that logic, we should only visit houses that needed painting and improve our odds to 100%. But Harry aspired to be a Supreme Court Justice and a commitment to balance was important to him. We would—or rather *he* would—knock on *all* doors. Our conversion rate over the summer ended up a little less than 1 percent, about the same as Diana's 5-year survival odds.

So what are the chances that a given prognosis is right? Supreme Court-aspirant Harry would say 50/50; it either is or it isn't. With the luxury of hindsight we could say either 0% or 100%; it either was or it wasn't. If that math doesn't make sense, it's because the question doesn't make sense. The nature of a prognosis makes the question irrelevant.

A medical prognosis, like any projected outcome—whether economic, political, personal, marital, environmental, or just about anything else—is essentially based on the following form:

1. Given what we know
    and
2. assuming nothing changes
    then
3. something is likely to happen.

But I think what we *don't* know is considerably more influential than what we *think* we do, so I'd assign a pretty low accuracy coefficient to the first step. And since change is constant and unavoidable, the second step completely invalidates the third so I find myself unable to invest much in the conclusion regardless of any caveats attached to it. To be honest, I'm having a very difficult time getting worked up about *any* prognostication these days, dire or otherwise.

There are, of course, legitimate concerns in the world that need attention, so is this just rationalization on my part to avoid being an agent of change in Step 2? Could be. Hard to know. But there's only been a single overriding issue that has affected my world for the past eight years. So is that just being selfish? You bet it is. But I'm clear about my role in the world right now and make no apology.

Diana's time was supposedly short, so we didn't spend much time worrying about long-term implications of anything. That is one of the ironic benefits of imminent death. We were guided by single-step cause-and-effect: we did whatever made Diana feel better immediately. There was no guessing about it. It either did or didn't. Is this approach sustainable? I don't know yet. I'll have to get back to you.

Diana's prognosis turned out to be both right *and* wrong. There's no question she has survived much longer that anyone anticipated. But on the other hand, at some point during that first three-to-twelve months Diana's life *did* end—and an even better one began.

The sun is up.
The sky is blue.

There's not a cloud to spoil the view. Summer in the Northwest can be spectacular. It might not get here until the first of August, but when it does, memories of a long winter become very short. The summer of 2006 came early and stayed late. My brother Tom and his family moved into the house next door, so now we had our own Lindsay Compound, like the Kennedys' Hyannis Port but without the money. We had the power, though—the Power of Loooooove.

Any member of our extended families who was able to travel made it to the island at some point during the summer. Local friends stopped by frequently and unannounced as did friends of friends and relatives of relatives and friends of relatives, possibly even people we didn't know. We often had a passel of babies and toddlers with unbound energy, elders with accumulated experience and wisdom, and every age in between to step in and step up with anything and everything they could do to help.

It was the inaugural All-Summer Games of Whidbey. We played golf. We played bocce. We played other ball games that hadn't yet been invented and which now we can't recall. We shucked oysters and dug for huge thick-necked clams called geoducks ("gooey ducks") that are 1) accessible only at extremely low tides, 2) profoundly tasty, and 3) somewhat obscene in appearance. We had taste tests of microbrews, single-malts, and—in

my favorite contest—one in which an unlabeled rum ran a close second for best Tequila in the sixth flight.

The summer was an open-ended party without a guest list. Anyone was welcome except, apparently, the tumor in Diana's left lung. It didn't seem fair, really, since we wouldn't have been having this gala if it weren't for her cancer in the first place, but fortunately the mass kept shrinking, like a wallflower 7th grader embarrassed to be at his own surprise birthday party. And like the insensitive 7th graders we likely were back in the day, we ignored it for the most part and went on dancing the night away. It was just too much fun being together.

So given all that, how is it even remotely possible that I could feel so lonely?

It turns out that loneliness is a common caregiver affliction regardless of how well supported we feel. In fact, for me, part of the loneliness was a direct *result* of all that support. I had to share Diana with everybody, almost all the time. I didn't really want to. I know, that's not even 7th grade; that's pre-school.

The worst part, though, was the loneliness even when no one else was around. The rope that was our life had unraveled, with the three strands of cord that were Diana, me, and everything we used to do together just lying there limp and frayed, running parallel instead of entwined. The synergy that provided strength and integrity was missing.

Diana was intent on fostering an internal dialogue with herself, and to help her do that she had rediscovered the primal language of music. She wanted to recapture some of the vitality of the young voice major she had been. She asked all of her friends for their favorite pieces of music, which she compiled into a meditation playlist. She would put on her headphones, lie back, close her eyes, and go… somewhere.

Decades ago, I decided to surprise our son Eric with a stop by the donut shop instead of driving straight to his preschool. I could see his growing consternation in the rearview mirror when he realized we had taken an unusual turn. "You know where we're going?" I asked, to which he solemnly replied: "No, but I know we're going somewhere my school *isn't!*"

Diana would go somewhere like that when she plugged into her iPod—somewhere I *wasn't.* I didn't begrudge her that. She needed to do it. But it left me by myself a lot. There were now extended periods that I could easily fill with mundane tasks and errands if I wanted to. But I didn't want to. I just wanted to be with her.

Everything I've ever learned about loneliness rode in on the AM airwaves of Country-Western radio. Nuthin' spells L-O-N-E-S-O-M-E like a three-legged dog in a pickup truck. A distillation of 40 years of Top 40 hits by Roy Acuff through Tammy Wynette clearly shows that loneliness involves some sort of abandonment by accident or design, either an actual or anticipated rejection through betrayal, being ditched, or even worse, just overlooked.

So working backwards: Was I being overlooked, ignored, or otherwise dismissed? Hmmm… not really. Not unless I wanted to be. Ditched? Diana went somewhere during her musical meditations, but I wasn't kept from trying to follow. Unless I chose to be excluded. Betrayed that Diana, a non-smoker would get terminal lung cancer? That's not betrayal. That's not even irony. Besides, who—or Who—would be the low-down no-good dirty double-crosser responsible for that betrayal? I've never found that a particularly helpful road to travel.

Well, dang me if it wasn't starting to look like my loneliness might just be self-inflicted. As a Country-Western theme, that's right up there with cheatin' hearts: somebody just stole my gal and now he's eyeing my self-pity.

By C&W standards I wasn't *lonely*; I was just *alone*. I've never really minded being alone and, in fact, sometimes I've preferred it. But while I had often *done* things alone—read, write, play, work—I wasn't used to just *being* alone with someone in the same room, especially someone I loved. I needed something to *do*. I needed... a hobby. It was time to pursue either 1) something I'd always thought I'd like to do but apparently not enough to actually try it, or 2) something I could do with a relatively inert woman listening to two centuries of classical music without bothering her.

Option #2 won out. I started giving Diana Jin Shin and other related energy treatments while she listened to her music. As Beethoven's deafness worsened, he relied on other faculties to "hear" his own music. I could almost hear him through my hands on Diana's body. We soon replaced external speakers with earbuds so we both could listen to the playlist. The effect on me was immediate and profound. I think the combination of the energy treatment and the music generated a waveform that doesn't reside in the conventional electromagnetic spectrum. It was like a carrier wave with a hidden coded message that gave directions to the healing place where Diana went. I had found my hobby.

Limbo

Recreationally, Limbo is one of those rare opportunities to succeed by actually lowering the bar. It is practiced by the invertebrate and the inebriate. Instead of bellying up to the bar, you belly under it, and regardless of the outcome, you typically end up on a Mexican beach with a cold cerveza, laughing. Nothing wrong with that. But that's not the Limbo that interests me.

Theologically, Limbo was neither Heaven nor Hell, out of God's hands and beyond the reach of Satan. It was a place reserved for the innocent and the ignorant, those oblivious to the concept of saving grace. Dante placed it in the suburbs, across the River Acheron from Downtown Hell. You could see the skyline, but not get there from here. I'm not a church guy. Very little religious dogma speaks to me, and practically none in a literal sense. But Dante is right on the money. The view into Hell from Limbo is spectacular.

Time has no meaning in Limbo. That's what makes it eternal. Eternity supposedly has no duration, but I've found that it does: it is 26.42 hours, the average time between Diana's CT scans and the appointment with the oncologist when we heard the results. That doesn't sound long, but it feels interminable. And Diana and I are among the lucky ones. The Seattle Cancer Care Alliance is extremely considerate of its patients. I've heard of other institutions where waiting for test results is measured in days or weeks, not hours. That's not interminable; that's criminal. That's not Limbo; that's full-contact fire and brimstone.

Based on the first few bi-monthly scans, we began to feel that

perhaps the main mass in Diana's lung had a short half-life, unlike Uranium and more like the last brownie in the pan. With each scan, only half of what was there previously remained. That's a pretty easy graph to plot. We got pretty excited. Limbo wasn't such a bad place after all, and actually started to feel something like Puerto Vallarta.

Right about then the tumor stopped shrinking.

Had we jinxed it? Well, if you believe in a fickle universe or a petulant god, then that's as good an explanation as any, but I suspect it's more complicated than that. We didn't know why it stopped shrinking, but then again, we didn't know why it *started* shrinking in the first place.

I'm not entirely clear on the statistics so I'll have to make this up: 97.6% of football teams that use the "prevent defense" to hang onto a slim lead end up losing the game. NFL, NCAA, high school, Pop Warner, sandlot, two-hand touch, or flag—it doesn't matter. It doesn't work for anyone. The idea behind this strategy is to stop doing what has worked for the entire game and start playing "safe." In West Texas, we called that being "yellow-bellied-chicken-livered." I have no idea why.

Had Diana and I seen the endgame too early and gone yellow-bellied-chicken-livered? Or were we just playing with less intensity? It was clear that something had changed, but what? Had the Tarceva stopped working? Had we slacked off on the Jin Shin? Were the blueberries for the smoothie being flown in from Peru instead of picked down the road? Had the Bee Gees snuck onto Diana's playlist? Had stress violated its restraining order?

Umm, well… yes, maybe, on that last one, especially. Diana was looking, acting, and feeling so much better that she had started feeling a little guilty about not carrying her weight in our company. Gravity, Gratitude, Guilt: that seems to be a natural progression in recovery. We had the great fortune of having extremely competent

and generous people in our company who had been filling Diana's considerable shoes with grace and good humor. But a perfect storm of events conspired to create a small gap in a project that only Diana could patch quickly and easily. And as projects always do, this one proceeded to regularly double in scope, the exact reverse of the half-life regression of Diana's tumor. This led to long hours and even longer plane rides. That led to sinus infections and pneumonia. Diana went to bed and I went ballistic.

Bad news, bitch, and blame. That's not so much a progression as it is a condition. I had a bad case. I knew it was unproductive, but I didn't appreciate at the time that it could be even more *counter*productive. I had been extremely vocal that Diana's working again wasn't healthy for her. Too soon. Too much. Too hard. But who's to say what caused her the most stress? The work, or my insistence that it was going to be bad for her? For that matter, who's to say it was stress? It could've been the Bee Gees.

I'd like to say I learned something about blame right then, but that is sadly not the case. I think the only cure for blame is perspective, and that only comes from experience, which my brother Targe says is what you get when you don't get what you want. I wanted Diana to get progressively better, a straight-line continuum to perfect health. But what I got was experience. And I was to get more and more of it as we went along.

So the tumor had stopped shrinking. That was the effect. There were innumerable candidates for the cause, and it was likely a chain of causes instead of a single one. So the answer to "Why?" is complicated. Sometimes I think the quickest and most obvious answer points to a question other than the one at hand, and "Why *that* question?" is the one that should be answered first. But one thing was clear. In the meantime, and until the next scan, we were back in Limbo.

Words fail me

Pulitzer Prize-winning Beat-era Zen-lumberjack Gary Snyder once said he wrote poetry because some things could be expressed no other way. That explains why many of us find some poems incomprehensible. My buddy Miles and I have discussed how words are often inadequate to the task of illuminating certain concepts, whether in prose or poetry. That's not necessarily a slight on our collective vocabulary; that's a failure of language itself. And to pull the thread a little further, I think there are even things that defy any conceptual framework whatsoever, for which both words and ideas not only fall well short, but actively erode understanding. Nothing has paid the price for that more than God.

In *Through the Looking Glass,* Humpty Dumpty tells Alice that he pays words extra if they work especially hard for him. Sometimes words don't work at all, but they do lie, cheat, and steal, often unintentionally. In those cases, Humpty may still pay them, but everyone else pays *for* them. I hate to think of the times I've misused words that meant the exact opposite of what I'd intended, words like "enervate" and "yes."

Sometimes it's better just to use an image; that's why we have international symbols for restrooms. But if a picture is worth a thousand words, then a metaphor can be worth ten times that many. Or it can be worth none. The exchange rate is difficult to track. Even so, allusions and metaphors don't cost much. They're an inexpensive way to cover matters that I would prefer not to spell out, whether because it would be too laborious or too painful.

So economical efficiency vs. cheap shortcut—that's the dichotomy and whether I view it as one or the other is largely a contest between perspective and patience.

The question in my mind when I gave Diana the Jin Shin Jyutsu treatments was: What exactly is the "energy" in "energy medicine" or "energy healing"? I could feel something tangible happening during the treatment. So could Diana. Both of us felt better afterwards than before. But we couldn't *quantify* anything—and that's the crux of scientific progress and verification: take a guess and measure whatever is measurable.

A brief summary of the scientific method, to which I heartily subscribe:

1. Hypothesize that something specific will occur under certain circumstances.
2. Design an experiment to measure something that tests the validity of Step 1.
3. Confirm, deny, or revise the hypothesis in Step 1 to account for all the data derived from the experiment in Step 2. Repeat as necessary or until the grant money runs out.

Actually, I left out the most important part: The Assumption. Developing a hypothesis in Step 1 is predicated on a specific worldview that represents the accumulated results of centuries of scientific method. This worldview is a moving target, so every hypothesis is derived from how we know the universe to be *now*. So there is no *correct* worldview, only a *current* worldview.

Asian cultures use words like "chi" and "prana" to refer to the active ingredient of these hands-on protocols, but they're both invariably translated as "energy" or "force" in their migration to the Western world. Unfortunately, the Western world knows how to

measure energy and force and nothing registers on equipment so finely tuned that it can tell which way a quark is facing deep within the Andromeda galaxy. If you can't measure it, does that mean it doesn't exist? Not exactly. Maybe we measured the wrong thing. Maybe what we want to measure can't be measured… yet. From a scientific point of view, having a hypothesis and being unable to test its validity is the same as having no hypothesis at all. It just doesn't contribute to figuring out how the universe works. It's not that the hypothesis is wrong; it's just that it doesn't matter.

The biggest problem I see is using the word "energy." It's a red herring the size of Moby Dick. Physicists have already laid claim to it. Besides, regardless of the topic I think it is a disservice to the thing itself to get bogged down in semantics, to get put off by a definition of what it may not in fact be. So I think of the word "energy" in this context as a metaphor, or at the very least a simile. In *Mama Makes Up Her Mind: And Other Dangers of Southern Living*, Bailey White writes about the desire for "something like a husband"—but what she really means is "exactly like a handyman." Whatever happens during a treatment I give Diana is probably "something like an energy" but very likely "exactly like something else"—but I have no idea what. It could be something we haven't yet seen, or an implication we haven't yet considered of something already discovered. Or it could be something not yet accommodated by the reigning worldview.

Almost all energy healing techniques have back stories about their origins and detailed explanations of the mechanisms by which they work. My issue… and it *is my* issue… is that I don't like any of them. I think they're entirely unnecessary and unhelpful. I'd love to be able to prove or even explain what happens during or as a result of a treatment to the satisfaction of an objective party and for the betterment of mankind, but I can't.

For me, whether Jin Shin Jyutsu worked or not wasn't a question of belief, but of disbelief. I didn't start to feel something between Diana and me during treatments because I started to *believe* that Jin Shin would work; I only felt it when I stopped insisting that it wouldn't.

Single-point perspective

It's commonly assumed that any catastrophic event in life somehow confers the superhuman ability to put things in proper perspective, to know what is truly important. I think it's more the case that any trauma (or non-trauma for that matter) offers the opportunity to consider a *different* perspective and ponder what *else* may be important, but *proper* perspective and *truly* important? Only if a radioactive spider is involved. Or a self-absorbed autocrat.

I can be as self-absorbed as the next autocrat. For me, knowing what was important has always been easy and self-evident: it was whatever I happened to be doing at the time. I readily accept that it may not be important to everyone—maybe not even *anyone*—else. That's the wonderful thing about importance in the era of self-esteem: everything falls into that category. So what if it's a subjective measure?

As an agent of change, catastrophe has a distinct advantage over routine daily life in its ability to radically alter context instantaneously. It's hard to know what's important when that catastrophe strikes, at least it was for me. So I thought about what was *un*important instead. We cancelled the newspaper. Then stopped cleaning the house. Missed bill payments. Deferred maintenance. Generally shirked responsibilities at work and in the community. It turns out that almost everything can fall just as well into the Unimportant category. There were, naturally, consequences to these inactions,

but they did clear a lot of stuff out of the way so that whatever was left must, by default, be important. For Diana, what was left standing was family. For me, what was left standing was Diana.

However, Diana and I shared a single goal: We each wanted to survive her cancer. Diana wanted to be able to live through it; I needed to be able to live with myself after it—regardless of the outcome. The only way for her to survive would be to follow her instincts and intuition. The only way for me to survive would be to follow her, to do whatever she wanted to do.

When I could set aside the likelihood of her dying, it turned out that it was a lot of fun doing whatever Diana wanted to do. Singular focus is not so much a discipline as it is a luxury. When Diana wanted to visit family, that's what we did. Our extended families are spread across the country. Some live in spectacular places, and we often had to pass through equally spectacular places on the way. When water became a prominent feature in Diana's dreams and meditations—cascading over her lungs and coursing among her cells—we visited every waterfall within 200 miles. We canoed the Stilliguamish, the Skykomish, the Snohomish, and the Sauk—rivers whose every cataract and syllable seemingly conferred some kind of healing power or protection. Then we'd ride the tandem bike we'd stashed downstream back to our car. If she visualized clean, crisp air filling her compromised lungs, we'd hike along the shoulders of the Cascades, walk the beaches of Puget Sound, or take in the breath of the old-growth forest just down the road.

That Diana felt well enough to even attempt any of these was the gift of a targeted chemotherapy that did minimal damage to her beleaguered immune system. That she became progressively stronger and more active as a result was a gift of living in the beautiful Northwest, the poster child for the Great Outdoors. That she was

becoming increasingly healthy while ostensibly dying was the gift of paradox, the patron saint of magicians and miracle workers.

Perspective is a funny thing. It's fleeting. Mercurial. Fickle. Half a degree one way or the other and it changes completely. As a standard of reference, it's overrated. I don't think a near-death experience yields any special insight or access to universal truths, and certainly no inviolate perspective. I don't claim any. But we did have an "Aha!" moment. It was the recognition that just prior to her diagnosis we had been wandering around in what could only be described as something approaching a near-life experience.

Slack tide

I t could be better. It could be worse. An optimist could utter either one of those statements. So could a pessimist. Without another point of reference, neither statement communicates anything other than a disregard for the present moment. Nothing we did leading up to and surpassing the one-year anniversary of Diana's diagnosis could entice the tumor to start shrinking again. Could've been better. But it wasn't growing, either, so it could've been worse. Projecting a trend is not so much about defining which parameters to consider as it is deciding which ones to ignore. That's why economic predictions are so variable—and so invariably worthless. Diana's tumor burden wasn't supposed to shrink in the first place, so the fact that it did for a period of time and then stopped shouldn't be something to get all worked up about. But we did anyway. At least for a little while. And then we moved on.

The poet William Stafford held himself to the discipline of writing a new poem every single day of his life. When asked how he felt about any given daily effort that didn't quite measure up, he simply replied, "Fine. I just lower my standards." That kind of practicality speaks to me. Diana maintained the highest of standards: to completely eliminate the cancer from her body. Zero. Zip. Nada. Mine were somewhat lower: maintain the status quo. That's because the status quo at that moment was pretty good. I didn't want the cancer to get worse, but it didn't have to get better, either. I started to think even terminal cancer might become a long-term manageable

disease, perhaps like diabetes, or political extremism.

Diana was from all outward appearances, healthy. Oh sure, she got pneumonia—but she recovered. You don't expect a Stage IV lung cancer patient who contracts a serious respiratory illness to survive intact and unimpaired, so that in itself was an indicator of good health in a qualified way. So the question was: How bad could it be if she felt so good? What were we to make of the absence of symptoms without medical imaging to reveal the status of the cancer? And conversely, what were we to make of a sudden shortness of breath? Or cough? What exactly is meaningful? What is trustworthy?

Our oncologist just laughed: "If you're feeling well, you're doing well." We were encouraged. We took that to mean there might be a way back from this. We just had to keep doing what we were doing. "Any pain?" he continued. There hadn't been for quite a while, but this time Diana reported that the back of her head was sore. That's not a good sign in a patient with a history of brain lesions. But this knot was from hitting her head on the crossbeam of the canoe when she was knocked backwards by a sweeper, a low branch overhanging the river that surprised us a day or two before. Our oncologist was visibly relieved. "You're so inspirational. Of all my patients, you're doing the most with the time you have left."

Ka-thunk.

We never asked outright, but it became clear that from an onco-logical view the future was undeniable, and still very dark. Despite Diana's exceptional progress the medical prognosis remained unchanged: This cancer would kill her. But until that day, "feeling well" was "doing well"—as in "as well as can be expected." I think we were less disturbed by his outlook than we were disappointed in it. We love our doctor for his experience and his good nature.

We are grateful for his top-ranked, leading edge facility. But like everything else, expertise has its limitations.

The distinction between hope and delusion is not a line in the sand, because that can be washed out by any sufficiently high tide. It's more like contested territory between opposing armies, a swathe of no-man's land that appears on the map at the sole discretion of whoever's drawing the chart. So if you find yourself in a similar situation, draw it yourself. The only time the line *might* exist in any real sense is in retrospect, so don't worry about getting it "right." Just be generous.

Smoke and mirrors

"I feel it in my fingers. I feel it in my toes. Love is all around me, and so the feeling grows." Nothing like a '60s love song by the Troggs. Unless it's another love song by the Troggs: *"Wild thing, you make my heart sing. You make everything grooooovy."* Maybe you had to be there.

By the end of the second summer, post-diagnosis, we were feeling extremely confident in Diana's prospects. The tumor in her left lung had stopped shrinking but was holding steady as of her last scan four months previously. All of the other areas of involvement—brain, pericardial effusion, mediastinal lymph nodes, and right lung—had by this time "resolved," which in the lexicon of radiology means "no longer of concern," which in patient language means "so then, they're gone, right?" And yes, that's what it means. It was oddly anticlimactic. We should have thrown them a going-away party.

But we were too busy partying ourselves. We decided to spend the day between the upcoming scan and the appointment to hear the results hiking with our good buddies Rene and Miles, so we piled into their car and headed east. Just before the Cascades run out onto the Columbia Plateau is the village of Leavenworth, not so much a part of Washington as it is a part of the Bavarian Alps, in much the same way as the Las Vegas Strip is representative of New York, Paris, or the Great Pyramid.

Half a century ago, Leavenworth was dying and desperate.

The sawmills had closed and the switching yard pulled up tracks and moved 20 miles east, hauling the community's livelihood with it. After languishing in the economic doldrums for a decade or so, the town started thinking not just outside the box, but outside the hemisphere, and recreated itself as a popular destination resort either quaintly bedecked in gingerbread or brazenly bewitched by crass commercialism, depending on how you look at it. And that's where we were headed.

However, we weren't going there for Leavenworth's schlock and schnitzel. We were there for its gateway into the Enchantments, a wilderness area of stunning and unrivaled beauty. We spent the afternoon hiking several miles up one side of Icicle Creek and back down the other, with a stop midway for brewed green tea on a slab of granite at the water's edge. Later we walked the banks of the Wenatchee River, which is both parallel to and worlds away from Main Street Leavenworth. All total, about seven miles hiking for the day along fast-flowing rivers, through sun-streaked meadows, and enveloped by the vanilla scent of Jeffrey pines. We spent the night in small rustic cabins that couldn't have been closer to the water had they been boats.

On the way back to Seattle, we invited Rene and Miles to the appointment with the oncologist so they could witness the tumor in full retreat for themselves. Diana was feeling so strong, so healthy, and so dynamic that we fully expected the scan to show the mass had disappeared altogether. We may have missed the chance to party when all the other areas of involvement had evaporated, but this was definitely going to be a time to celebrate. We could feel it in our fingers. We could feel it in our toes.

What we couldn't feel was it growing in her lung.

"How is this possible?" was the second question I asked myself after the oncologist gave us the news. (The first, I'm ashamed to

say, was "How many times do I have to go through this?") This was hardly any different than the original diagnosis, maybe even worse, which, of course, is the big downside of Hope. Don't get your hopes up or you might be disappointed. It's far easier—and infinitely more tragic—to just start disappointed and stay there. So how many times do I have to go through this? As is often the case, I had asked myself the wrong question. The real question was, "Why do I react like this?" Because this won't be—and perhaps still isn't—the last time the tumor will grow.

As to how the tumor could possibly be growing when we were doing everything "right"? Well … I think it's still possible to be right, but maybe about the wrong thing. How we spent each day—the smoothies, hands-on treatments, walking, being outdoors, minimizing stress, enjoying our time with friends and family—may not by itself be the cure for cancer, or even the key to living long, but it was certainly instrumental to living well. And living well might be as much as we could—maybe even *should*—hope for.

But if curing the cancer was indeed to be the goal, it would apparently require something more. For that, we'd have to take our cue from a deathbed railroad town that reinvented itself as an unfathomably popular Bavarian resort, an enchantment that rivals its adjacent pristine wilderness. I had always gotten hung up on the kitsch—and still do—but that's hardly the point. The impressive part of Leavenworth's resurrection is not how close it's come to the real Bavaria, but how far it had to go to get there.

Diana and I would have to do something similar. We would have to reinvent ourselves, to *reimagine* ourselves. And this was when things started to get a bit… interesting.

Lack of vision quest

When I think about crossroads of significance in our life—opportunities that sent us in a direction other than the way we were headed—the decisions were invariably based not on there being a good reason for doing something in particular, but on there being no particularly good reason *not* to.

Mid-September of 2007 found us wading through the aftermath of the news that the mass in Diana's left lung was growing again. She had talked the oncologist out of traditional chemotherapy and into trying another type of highly targeted radiation similar to the one used on her brain lesions. This was considered experimental and unproven for use on lung tumors, but the radiologist was optimistic. The treatment date was still two weeks away when a friend casually mentioned: "I know a good medicine man…"

Our subsequent visit to an authentic Muckleshoot tribal shaman wasn't an act of desperation; it was just an exploration into the previously unconsidered, and there was no particularly good reason not to. I had absolutely no idea what to expect. That was a good thing, since the entire evening, from the time we left Seattle to the time we got back, was a series of wonderfully inventive non sequiturs with no apparent common thread.

The shaman didn't live in a hogan or a tipi, as it turned out. Nor was he a hermit, or wearing anything special to denote that

he was the sacred and spiritual link to anyone who crossed the Bering Strait during the last Ice Age. I didn't expect that he would be, though, so I wasn't disappointed.

While Diana was outside with the shaman, a blue plastic tarp sheltering them from the drizzle, I remained in the family room of his suburban rambler with people waiting to be treated. Here the shaman's Caucasian wife carried on with one story after another, each one plumbing greater depths of inanity; the stepson chimed in with examples of misguided forays into the world of electricity; the surly stepdaughter, headphones intact, walked two steps into the room before noticing us all, sneered, and left; two yippy dogs ran around, sniffing and shedding; cats roamed, slept, and rubbed against our legs; the young devout Christian couple waiting to be treated clutched the Bible they brought as their required "offering," and I watched their eyes widen as it dawned on them that offerings typically get burned. The pall of incense, scented candle, or maybe dinner hung in the air and there I sat, mired in the mundane and meaningless, while Diana and the shaman were outside in the rain and domain of solemn ritual.

What was up with these people? Could this actually be happening? And then it occurred to me that perhaps it wasn't. What if I treated this like a dream? How would I interpret this cast of characters, this non-series of events? Well… pretty easily, as it turned out. Each represented something that would ordinarily trigger irritation in me. And here they all were in one room, at one time. If I were indeed asleep, this wouldn't be a dream; it would be a nightmare.

And that's when I woke up. The thing that was wrong with this picture was… *me*: everything belonged in the shaman's family room except the arrogant and judgmental guy with the attitude.

My buddy Randy tells the story about the man who spends

all of his money and most of his time seeking the meaning of life. When he finally arrives at the mountaintop, the yogi tells him "Life is a river." The man is incredulous—and furious. He yells, "After all I've been through, you're really going to just sit there and give some simplistic, sophomoric platitude about Life being a river?" The yogi is taken aback: "You mean life *isn't* a river?"

I kinda like Life being a river. We'd canoed down too many that summer to not notice the parallels. But now I'm thinking the river isn't the metaphor—*Life* is the metaphor. Sometimes Life is just too weird to be real. I think the evening with the shaman was actually meant for me, not Diana. Homeopathic remedies expose you to a minute sample of what's making you sick in order to cure you. This was homeopathy on steroids.

Now when events conspire to put me in the exact place I'm trying to avoid, or when the bizarre strikes unbidden for no apparent reason, I try not to think of these things as happening *to* me, but *for* me. Then it's just a matter of figuring out the what of it, not the why.

You would not believe how much easier this has made daily life. I take fewer things personally and even fewer things irritate me. Someone cuts me off on the freeway? I don't even honk: I know the bastard's just a metaphor. And if it's something a bit more serious and drawn out, something like my wife having terminal cancer? Well, that falls into the realm of allegory. Those can be a bit tricky. It takes longer to work those out.

Ready or not...

What in other circumstances could have been a memorable romantic moment cuddled up in the big leather chair in the living room at midnight devolved into just a memorable moment when Diana, recovering from a punctured lung and curled up post-operatively on my lap in her robe, passed out and threw up at exactly the same time. Just as I was trying to extricate both the vomit from her throat so she could breathe and my heart from mine so I could scream for help, she woke up, slightly confused but entirely convinced that *I* was the one having the health crisis.

This type of fainting spell is called a vasovagal episode. She'd had one during the surgery several days prior, to implant gold BB's that would be tracked by the machine targeting her radiation treatment later in the week. I'd listened carefully to the hospital discharge orders that mentioned the possibility of other vasovagal episodes. I already knew that pain—as well as many pain meds—can cause nausea, and I had been trained as a First Responder in a volunteer fire department. So you could say I was prepared for the event that evening, in the same sense that a trussed-up pork loin rubbed in olive oil and Herbs de Provence is "prepared" for what's coming next. No manual had ever addressed the possibility that the dead weight of a person half my size would pin me to a cushy chair, effectively rendering me useless.

Be Prepared. Robert Baden-Powell, the founder of the Boy Scouts, chose a motto to match his monogram. When asked

"*Prepared for what?*" he reputedly replied, "*Why, for any old thing!*" That explains why merit badges are so numerous and varied, even though most have been superseded by iPhone apps.

Is it even possible to be prepared for anything that comes up? Based on my performance that evening, knowledge and training were easily trumped by circumstance. Personal experience fares no better. You'd think Diana's early-stage colon cancer in 1993 would've better prepared me for her late-stage lung cancer in 2006, but it was hardly even a training exercise. Back then it had been three surgeries, a temporary colostomy, and six months later we were back to business as usual. I didn't learn anything to prepare me for the next time. But Diana passing out, puking, and pinning me to the chair? Now I know to sit on *her* lap.

The only times that I've really felt prepared in my life were in areas or on occasions that interested me. I've found curiosity to be a better motivator for readiness than fear or worry. Worst-case scenarios too often insinuate themselves into and subsume otherwise-benign actual events. Hypothetical situations, on the other hand, are nowhere near as self-fulfilling but only because they are notoriously simplistic in scope, rarely imitating the complexity of available options in real life. They contribute to paranoia, not preparedness.

Sometimes the best preparation for something is to not be burdened by something else: preoccupation, surprise, doubt, fear, elation… The problem for me, historically, is not feeling that I had to know what to do in any given situation, but closing the gap between recognizing that something has indeed occurred and doing something about it, i.e., squeezing the I-can't-believe-this-is-happening middleman. The question of how, what, or why—and even whether any of them are correct—is becoming less important to me than the when.

Merit badges notwithstanding, I can't help but think Baden-Powell intended his *"Be Prepared... for any old thing"* as a means, not an end. Preparedness is not what I know or how I know it. It isn't the product of skills, knowledge, and experience plotted on a scale with *Reaction Time* as one axis and *Hope That Doesn't Happen* the other. I think he meant it as "Be Prepared... for any old thing *could* happen." It is simply an acknowledgement that both opposition and opportunity exist within the inherent and inevitable changes of a lifetime. I don't think he meant "Be Prepared [for something specific]" but "Be Prepared [for Life]." In other words, not "Brace Yourself," but *"Em*brace Yourself."

Next stop: The Twilight Zone

The waiting room during Diana's first surgery for colon cancer in 1993 was crowded with family and friends. Some needed to be there to assuage their own worries and to lend their presence for Diana's benefit. A few were there because they needed support themselves, but most, I suspect, were there because they felt I needed the support, so that I should be distracted from the consequences and implications of what was going on behind the swinging doors.

So they essentially threw a surprise party without the guest of honor, with the high-level chatter of friends who hadn't seen each other for awhile overlying the low-level hum of anxiety that was all the more obvious because of the intense effort to dispel it. I loved them all, but I hated it. It's my party and I'll cry if I want to.

I didn't really cry. I just left.

Almost every hospital has what used to be called the "Chapel" but is often now just the "Quiet Room." It only mattered to me that it was away from the party—and small. This one doubled as storage for extra chairs and boxes, but I was only interested in solitude, not sanctity. I straddled a metal folding chair, rested my head on my arms, closed my eyes, and went to work.

The surgical waiting room is the only time and place in a clinical setting where Diana and I have been apart during any of her health issues, and if I can't be *with* her, I want to be thinking

about her. I certainly don't want to be distracted *from* her. So I began going through the surgical procedure in my head, step by step, from administering the general anesthetic through the incision and excision to the "close 'er up." All this took about five minutes because I'll admit to being a little vague on the specifics. I found myself relying on a childhood memory of the internal organization of the Invisible Woman® Human Body model but, frankly, there were other body parts that had interested my 5th-grade self more than the large intestine.

During the rest of the surgery I pictured myself as a miner with a headlamp and an array of tools painstakingly chipping away at a large, malignant mineral deposit protruding from a cave wall. I was meticulous. No errant crystal or flake escaped the reach of my pick, broom, and shovel. By the end of the two hours I had eleven-and-a-half ore carts filled with debris, ready to be hauled away. At that point, someone tapped me on the shoulder and told me the surgeon was in the waiting room.

Flash forward fourteen years to early October, 2007. We were in the CyberKnife stereotactic radiosurgery suite in the basement of Swedish Medical Center in Seattle. The radiologist was going to try to kill Diana's growing tumor using some 200 carefully spaced and targeted beams from a particle accelerator, a smaller version of the Large Hadron Collider in Switzerland that would later be used to discover the elusive subatomic particle that holds the universe together. A much, much smaller version.

Diana underwent a 90-minute treatment three days in a row in which she had to remain almost perfectly still. To help her do this she loaded up all of our friends' favorite pieces of music onto her iPod, four-and-a-half hours worth. The only criterion? It shouldn't make her want to dance.

When they took Diana away to the treatment room, I was left

alone in the waiting room. Really alone. My only companions were a stylish sofa, a ceramic planter filled with bamboo, and a wall tank of fish from an alien world. I had loaded up Diana's extended playlist onto my own iPod and decided we'd listen to the same thing she was while under the ray gun just 20 feet away. I plugged in, straightened up, and closed my eyes.

Within the first few bars of the first piece, I found myself standing in the middle of Pine Valley, a beautiful meadow deep within the Ventana Wilderness Area of California where Diana and I would've gotten engaged had I not decided that the dusty, poorly lit basement of our dorm was more romantically suited for a proposal a day later. At first only Diana and I were in the meadow. With each successive piece of music more people arrived, each apparently taking their cue from whatever was playing.

Eventually, I think everyone Diana and I ever knew together or separately showed up. People from her past I'd never met; some from mine I could barely recall; many who have been important to us, but with whom we have since lost touch; and more than a few I had no expectation, or even interest, in ever seeing again—all of us laughing, talking, or standing with our arms around each other in the '60s Sway, depending on the song. This was not a distraction; this was a celebration. This was Diana's "Love-in" on a much larger stage, on which Joe Cocker belted out "With a Little Help from my Friends" as fireworks and spotlights illuminated the sky from Salinas to Tassajara.

Tears were streaming down my face when Diana emerged from the treatment room. So what had *she* experienced during the session? Well, within the first few bars of the first piece of music, she found herself standing in the middle of Pine Valley, the beautiful meadow deep within the Ventana Wilderness Area of California where...

I knew the make-believe miner during the colon surgery years earlier had emerged from my imagination. I had directed his every move, scripted every grunt. That was realistic, not real. But the meadow? I didn't direct any of that. It just unspooled on its own. And it was as real as anywhere I've ever been. Did Diana and I experience the same moments at exactly the same time? Who knows. Probably not. No way to tell. But it was eerily synchronous when we compared notes over dinner, especially when we got to Joe Cocker. I can't explain what happened; I can only acknowledge that it did.

I've been in more than a few waiting rooms. Each one is the same in its own unique way. Whether it's a folding chair in a hallway, an institutional room with the plastic ambiance of a McDonald's, or a well-appointed retreat that follows the dictates of Feng Shui or Wabi-Sabi, they all suffer from the same fundamental affliction: they shouldn't be called "Waiting" rooms. I consider them points of departure, as exotic and mysterious as any depot along the Orient Express, portals to the unexplored reaches of inner space, metaphysical transports that allow me to be in two places at once—where I have to be and where I need to be.

Waiting
and seeing

There are five types of desert in the American Southwest: Chihuahuan, Sonoran, Mojave, Big Basin, and Cultural—the range of this last one coinciding with the city limits of Las Vegas. From the middle of any of the other four on a cloudless night of a new moon, far removed from the ambient light cast by semis and suburbs, the sky seems to be filled with every star in the universe, and each one is within reach. Distances collapse. Time dissolves. The cold expanse of interstellar space becomes intimate and reveals why myths, legends, and love poems find their origins in those winking, welcoming points of light, those angels and lost souls, those pinpricks of unrelenting and remorseless radiation.

To extrapolate from Ronald Reagan's ill-advised and insensitive comment about redwoods, "If you've seen one star, you've seen 'em all." True enough, but only if viewed with the unaided eye since by that standard each one simply looks like an undifferentiated circle of white nothingness. The human eye just can't detect the subtleties of the electromagnetic scale. No need to feel bad, though, because neither can a multimillion-dollar Computed Tomography scanner.

An irradiated body part apparently remains too "hot" to get an accurate assessment of treatment efficacy for six months. And indeed the CT scan taken three months after Diana's stereotactic radiosurgery looked like an infrared aerial photograph of the fire bombing of Dresden. *Everything* was lit up: the treatment area,

surrounding tissues, and the various flight plans the individual beams had followed to reach their target. I wondered why we had bothered to bombard Diana's lung with one type of x-ray just to get an inconclusive evaluation of the effects of another. "Can't really tell anything from this," reported the radiologist, "but it's looking good. It's just what we expected to see." See? Or *not* see?

So we geared up to wait another three months to let the radioactive dust settle and find out if the tumor was really sincerely dead, or just sorta dead. No big deal. It wasn't as though we had to put our life on hold while we waited.

As a matter of fact, life went on at an accelerated pace in many respects. We welcomed a brand-new grandson into the world, and helped his older sister negotiate her way through a brand-new world of her own. We tagged along on the artistic coattails and intellectual lapels of our multitalented children and their spouses: presentations of papers at academic symposia; premieres of pieces in concert halls; exhibitions of artworks in shows and galleries. We would light out in search of fun in the sun, but just as likely get pneumonia as a tan. We would return home to the stormy skies of the Northwest and the rumblings of impending discord in our extended family that would cloud the future in coming months. Most of this was exhilarating; some exhausting; often both. In some ways, it was a brand-new world for us, too.

For me at the time, there was nothing effortless about waiting. Just the idea of waiting created an apparent vacuum where none actually existed. Opportunities and obligations rushed in to claim territory like white settlers in the Oklahoma Land Run, much to the chagrin of the Shawnee and Cheyenne. A change of ownership was involved in my case, too. For some inexplicable reason, upon the bugle blast of the radiation treatment I effectively transferred responsibility for Diana's and my well-being to the Western medical community.

Almost everything I had been doing and feeling really good about—the hands-on treatments, adventures outdoors, forays into the mysterious world of Eastern thought, exclusive focus on Diana—was subsequently, gradually, almost imperceptibly displaced with each passing day until it was conveniently confined to a reservation in the Black Hills of South Dakota. Why would I do this? Well… because it was easier, for one thing, but the real reason was because I had obviously not yet discovered the gold in them thar Black Hills.

There is a two-lane highway in the middle of Nevada that runs through the Great Basin desert and hasn't seen traffic since the last wagon train. Driving that stretch at night is the closest I'll ever come to the suspended animation of intergalactic flight, nothing but stars ahead of me and behind. By day the distance between two points is measured in gallons and it's easy to be seduced by single-point perspective. I know I've arrived when the road ends. In the meantime, it can take some effort to look away from the painted white line and off to the side, where the base of the hills in the distance has been lightly sprayed with a thin purple mist.

It takes even more effort to actually pull over. And get out. And walk over to see what has the audacity to mar a perfectly drab landscape with a splash of color. The nondescript magenta flowers are spaced as far apart as the stars in the heavens and just as numerous. Up close they're miniscule; from the road a mirage, a conspiracy of light, angle, season, and happenstance. Like most things, the singular effect is far removed from the possible cause—whether one among many or many in concert—and that is why it typically takes a myth, or a legend, or a love poem to connect them. It's easy to miss and hard to appreciate something like that at 80 miles per hour, even when on a parallel path.

War zone

The radiosurgical strike on Diana's tumor had met its objective. Accurate targeting. Acceptable collateral damage. Minimal loss of lifestyle. We celebrated, of course, but stopped short of unfurling a "Mission Accomplished" banner, not because we were doubtful of the results but because you just never know if heavy-handed hubris is going to turn around and slap you silly. Six months after treatment the scan showed just a small irregular-shaped white blob with nothing growing on or around it, like the Bikini Atoll after the H-bomb tests. "We got what we were aiming at," the radiologist crowed. "What we're seeing is likely just scar tissue."

So all quiet on the upper lobe, which meant I could turn my attention to another theater of operations: the skirmish between the hospital and the insurance company. We were extremely lucky to have 1) access to leading medical technology, and 2) a good insurance policy. They served well together. We were proud of both of them. But now they had wandered into disputed territory. The stereotactic radiosurgery was a bit *too* leading-edge for our carrier. While the procedure was approved for use on the brain, it did not have a proven track record in the lung. That categorized it as "Experimental," which in the arcane dialect of Health Coverage Fine Print meant "Excluded."

Every standard medical protocol was at one time considered experimental. Unfortunately, so was every medically catastrophic failure. For the insurance industry, the task is to identify the point *not* when the proposed procedure becomes warranted and reasonable

from a patient's point of view but from the perspective of payout vs. profitability. For that analysis they need data. There wasn't any. The practice was too new. The insurance company denied the claim, but offered the possibility of appeal. The burden of proof therefore lay with me, not them.

Diana was a sample size of one. That the treatment apparently worked for her wasn't proof enough. I needed more data points. So where did I go for data that didn't exist? Google, of course, the magic portal to raw, unfiltered information that has as good a chance of being sorta true and kinda accurate as not. Maybe.

I worked on the appeal somewhat haphazardly over several months. I located some published studies, but most were either funded by or performed at the behest of the manufacturer of the radiological equipment in question. I was thrilled when I finally came across references to several blogs of other patients who had had the same exact treatment on their lungs the previous year. I clicked one of the links. The page had been renamed "In Loving Memory..." The next blog had also been reworked: "In Memoriam..."

I had stepped into a minefield. I stopped following links. I stopped working on the appeal. I just... stopped. I could not go forward and the only way to retrace my steps was to figure out how I got there. And why.

I had barreled down the appeal path without even thinking about it. The denial of claim hadn't been a complete surprise, but the hospital's ineffectiveness in overturning it on our behalf had been. So I'd taken up the flag myself—to try to get out of paying for something after-the-fact that I'd been more than willing to gut our retirement fund to pay for beforehand.

It wasn't that I objected to the way I was spending my time on the appeal, but rather the way I was spending my mind. I resented the insidious way that fear and doubt had wormed under the barbed

wire and infiltrated my conscience and confidence. It was unseemly and unnecessary. We had already decided well in advance that the cutting-edge, minimally invasive treatment for Diana would be worth whatever it cost. Just the *possibility* that it would work was what made it worthwhile; the apparent success was a bonus. On the other hand, making the case for the appeal was turning out to be maximally invasive for me. While the medical procedure itself was costly, the appeal process was even more so. I let the appeal deadline come and go.

Ultimately, the hospital offered to split the remaining difference on the bill, which I gratefully accepted. I told Diana about that part, but very little about the rest. At the time I had just said it was hard to make the case for the appeal. I didn't say what made it hard. Diana will find out about the memorial websites when she reads this. My ambivalence about the curiosity cabinet of wonders that is the Internet will finally make sense to her. And someday—if we're really lucky and everything goes well—she'll find out about our new improved retirement plan: huddled together in a flimsy single-wide trailer on the outskirts of Tijuana. Far better that than the old plan still intact and me living in our beautiful home alone.

Weight! Weight! Don't tell me...

There are examples in Western literature of love so profound that the death of one party is followed shortly thereafter by the death of the other from heartbreak. It is a sub-genre of Romantic Tragedy not nearly as popular as it could be only because, frankly, it is a commercial dead-end. There is no *Romeo & Juliet II*.

However, the mythology endures. Diana and I adopted it early on in our marriage, when it was still safe to do so. So, apparently, had Diana's maternal grandparents. GrantiPop died of a heart attack just weeks shy of Grandmother's death from lung cancer. But they had lived a good life together, and they were soooo old. They were at least… let's see… a few years younger than I am now.

So the parallels were a bit troubling. Was I going to die right after Diana? And perhaps even worse by literary standards: if I didn't, had I not loved her enough? Given her grandparents' sterling example, Diana had her own misgivings: GrantiPop died first under the burden of taking care of Grandmother. Was I, therefore, going to keel over *before* Diana did, whenever that might be?

These were not our foremost questions in the Spring of 2008 but they had been hiding in there among the lesser concerns for quite some time. I was not GrantiPop, however. I felt no obligation to follow his example, but there was a small voice chained to the wall in my dungeons that weakly whimpered, "If Diana goes, why bother?" So I didn't pay much attention to my own health—violating

rule numero uno for caregivers—and I indeed started to look like overweight, out-of-shape GrantiPop, while Diana didn't look like she was going to follow Grandmother through the veil anytime soon. This presented a significant problem for both of us, though I did my best to ignore it.

My exercise programs and history closely parallel the life cycle of a slime mold: a period of intense, frenetic motility followed by a much, much longer period that is unequivocally sedentary. Diana tentatively pointed this out to me when we were out for dinner as I vegetated in front of a platter of deep-fried everything. I acknowledged this conversation-stopper with the same grace of any other overweight, middle-aged guy: I was pissed.

And so began a period of enlightenment. I am fortunate to possess tremendous will power, except when I don't. Spite has historically been a motivator for me, I'm sorry to say, so I put on the pedometer Diana gave me two Christmases previously—a gift that was way too subtle for me at the time—and I stopped eating obvious junk, which turned out to be a surprisingly significant percentage of my diet.

I also started eating half-sized portions with half-sized bites chewed twice as long. I felt better within a week, and really pretty good within two. I'd dropped maybe 30 pounds the first month, as we aimed for and often exceeded by far the recommended 10,000 steps per day. There would be times when I couldn't feel any weight on the soles of my feet, as if I were walking a straight line through the twisted streets of Seattle's Tangletown neighborhood with the world turning this way and that to accommodate my path at every corner. While the muscle tone of my underworked body and overwrought heart hadn't exactly returned, it was at least within shouting distance.

My mantra became "mobility, agility, and flexibility" in body,

mind, and spirit. I felt all kinds of weight—physical, mental, psychic, literal, metaphorical, imaginary—lifted from me, a transformation that had started with Diana's hesitant comment over bar food. It took me months before I thanked her for it, though. I *think* I thanked her. Maybe not. Could be there's an infinitesimally small part of me that's still pissed. Transformative doesn't necessarily mean transcendent.

Uncertainty 98249

When pulled over for speeding and asked if he knew how fast he was going, Nobel laureate Werner Heisenberg replied, "No, but I know where I am." That joke apparently leaves freshman physics students rolling in the aisles of the lecture hall at MIT. I had to have it explained to me. It has to do with electrons. You can know either the velocity of an electron or its location, but not both. If you know one, you can only speak of the other in probabilities. It's not a question of measurement accuracy, but a fundamental characteristic of matter. Into a mechanistic view of the universe rooted in Isaac Newton's apple tree, Heisenberg introduced the concept of Uncertainty as a scientific principle.

This same principle comes into consideration when planning the course of a radiation treatment. Blanket the area where the cancer might be going? Or focus precisely on the area where it definitely is right now? Not an easy choice. Radiological oncology may hail from the ivory tower of academic pursuit, but it deals in the underworld of trade-offs, guesses, and gambles. Sometimes it comes up sevens and elevens; sometimes snake-eyes.

"That was outside the area we treated," the radiologist told us, pointing at a small undistinguished maybe-something that had appeared on Diana's scan in June 2008, nine months after the highly targeted stereotactic treatment. "We got everything in the target region."

That may even have been true. But it hardly mattered.

"We won't know if it's anything for a couple of months when we take another scan," continued the radiologist. "How comfortable are you with uncertainty?"

We were relatively unfazed by this news, and that surprised us more than the appearance of the blot on the scan. But this was no longer foreign territory. We had been there before. We knew the customs. We knew the language. We knew what to expect. I wasn't comforted by that, but I wasn't discomfited, either. That didn't mean I had become a fatalist. Or a realist, for that matter. I think I was an uncertainist, but that was a relatively recent development.

I have historically been uneasy with ambiguity. That probably stems from my Presbyterian upbringing with our 1) collective belief in predestination, and 2) absolute confusion about what that means. To my adolescent ears it sounded like, maybe damned if you do, maybe damned if you don't, maybe damned even if you forgot the question. God knows ahead of time (that's the "pre" part) but I won't find out until it's too late (that's the "destination" part). That is uncertainty at its most definite.

Consequently—or maybe coincidentally—I have always felt more comfortable once I knew the lay of the land. If I could have only one of the 10 Essentials of Wilderness Travel, I'd choose the map every time. I'd rather find myself up the creek than in the dark. So here we were, back in the doctor's office facing the possibility that Diana's 2nd primary cancer in 12 years was growing for the 3rd time. Why was I not reacting badly? I think because by that time I'd finally pieced together that when it comes to the terrain of cancer, uncertainty *is* the lay of the land.

Our oncologist suggested, "Let's wait and see what the next scan tells us. Just put it out of your mind until then." Surprisingly, Diana and I then saw that insignificant little blur on a CT scan for what it really was: an opportunity. The little smudge rematerialized

not as a focal point, but a point of departure, a course correction. Unlike Heisenberg and his electrons, we knew neither where we were nor where we were going. You might think that would be a disadvantage, but it was surprisingly liberating.

What we *did* know was where we'd been. Since the radiation treatment nine months before, we had resolutely and exclusively stayed the course charted by Western medicine. But it hadn't felt right. It was time to recalibrate our compass. Diana would continue to spend two seconds of each day swallowing the targeted chemo pill because… well, why not? And for that very same reason we'd devote the rest of our waking hours to exploring the ancient and anecdotal avenues of the Far Elsewhere.

So to answer the radiologist's question about how comfortable we had become with uncertainty: Very. We had listed it as our home address on the last census. We had come for the cancer but stayed for the climate. Uncertainty is a thriving and supportive expatriate community open to those of any former persuasion. We'll likely retire here. So whenever any card-carrying residents of *Certainty* inadvertently wander through… well, I may or may not entertain them, but I *will* try my best to humor them.

Total immersion

When Diana was 13, her family pulled up roots and relocated to Switzerland. She and her younger siblings were abruptly thrown into the local school system, and while all four came home the first day in tears, at least they were crying in French. I, too, was transplanted into a foreign culture at an early age when my family abandoned drought-stricken West Texas for the fecund Central Valley of California, where my brothers and I had to trade Real American for Proper English.

It's not just learning a foreign language that benefits from total immersion. It also works for religion, which might explain why the solemn Presbyterian sprinkling on my forehead as a baby didn't really register. But if you full dip a fervent Pentecostal in the symbolic River of Jordan, he comes up sputtering in Tongues. Sometimes you just need a good dunking to do it right.

The hands-on treatments I'd been giving Diana were based on whatever I'd gleaned from books and friends, or anything I might have intuited while doing them. I had not been formally trained in any of the methods. It was like wading in the shallows of a clear, cold mountain lake with the water lapping a bit North of my knees and just South of my… commitments. If Diana and I were going to resolve the little blot that had showed up on her scan using means other than additional medical intervention, I was going to have to man up and go deeper.

At heart, I am an observer. In the wings, on the sidelines, behind the camera. I typically stand back and watch… consider…

calculate. And then from the safety of the shadows I either 1) offer insightful commentary, or 2) take a cheap shot. Being in the thick of it has no appeal to me. In most debate I try to maintain a certain professional distance and objectivity, which can also be referred to as "being a chicken-shit" in the vernacular of Real American. It's also called that in Proper English. I don't know what it is in French.

So it was time to ditch the water wings. I decided I had to get some bona fide training in one of these hands-on energy methods. But which one? I felt indebted to Jin Shin Jyutsu since that was what started us down this road, but the seminars were five days long and several states distant. I didn't want to be away from Diana that long, or away from the $895 at all. Healing Touch and acupressure presented similar obstacles. The only modality that was local, short, and inexpensive was something called Reiki, which I'd read about and had already tried to incorporate into Diana's treatments. Reiki also appealed to my generalist tendencies, since it seemed to involve just the seven chakras instead of the 26 points used in Jin Shin and the hundreds used in acupressure. So cheap-and-easy won the day.

A Reiki class is typically a one-day affair for $125 or so, which includes a series of "attunements" by a Reiki Master that you obviously cannot get from a book. I came across a flyer for a Reiki class being offered the very next weekend just five miles from home. Across the top was written: "Using Reiki On Your Garden Fairies."

I was ready for the Reiki. I wasn't ready for the fairies. At least not then. These days I cannot categorically deny the existence of fairies or anything that might be mistaken for them or acting on their behalf, but I can assure you there are obviously none in our garden regardless of their actual existence or their need for Reiki.

I looked further afield and located a Reiki introductory class in Bellevue, about an hour away across the ferry. A week later I walked

into a classroom that had soft music, tea, a circle of chairs, and the same vibe as the '70s personal growth workshops against which I'd sealed my mind with a curse to rival Ramses.

"This is never going to work," I told my Knee-Jerk Inner Skeptic.

"I know!" he laughed. "What a joke!"

"No, I mean it's never going to work with you here," I replied.

And with that I consciously, deliberately, and completely relaxed my mind, allowing all the toxic prejudice, objections, and misgivings to drain out through the soles of my feet, across the floorboards, down the pavement, and into the storm sewers of Bellevue that empty into Lake Washington where the EPA has no jurisdiction. And then I was ready to experience the class for whatever it was, at entirely face value.

Very little of the content was new, and while I approached the first attunement with some curiosity, my expectations were neutral at best. It was performed with appropriate ceremony, our eyes closed, the room quiet. I could feel the Reiki Master do something around my head and then blow sharply through my pressed palms toward my forehead. *What the hell was that*? The puff of air penetrated my skull and into my brain an inch and a half. It felt like one of those pneumatic prods used to put down cattle in Chicago stockyards, but nonlethal—except to my Knee-Jerk Inner Skeptic, who promptly drowned in Lake Washington.

Reiki is a Japanese system that dates back a hundred years, with roots that go back several millennia more. It's based on the idea of a universal life force that pervades everything and everywhere. Someone who has been "attuned" can act as a conduit through which the person being treated draws and uses that life force to heal himself or herself. Therefore a Reiki practitioner is not a healer; the recipient is the healer. That's the short version.

Does it really work that way? *Beats me.* Does it work at all?

Yes, it does. Do I care to elaborate on that? *No, I don't.* Don't or won't? *Can't.*

So I had waded in way, way over my head. Or maybe I'd waded in without my head. Either one is apt. In the weeks that followed the class I would find myself at times madly treading water to keep from sinking, at other times floating on my back watching the sky gently spin, and occasionally sitting on the bottom, a gilled and gilded Buddha with a weight belt.

The reason the world looks different from the middle of a lake than from the shore is because the world *is* different from there. Unfamiliar and unexpected. Exhilarating and exotic. Remote and refreshing. It was actually a very good place for me to be. I had a lot to not think about. Even more to not talk about. Learning a language that doesn't exist can be a bit of a challenge, even when fully immersed.

Sense and nonsense

Several years ago we visited the asylum in San Remy that harbored Vincent van Gogh while he worked out some personal issues and hoped his ear would grow back. Looking through the flawed and inconsistent thickness of glass in the windows overlooking the fields and courtyard turned the olive trees, mown hay, benches, walkways, and people into undulating, indistinct versions of themselves, just like… a van Gogh painting. The heretical thought occurred to me that perhaps van Gogh wasn't always painting his impressions or interpretations, but what he literally saw.

Perceptions are funny things. We depend on them to discover the apparent workings of the world and to fix our place in it. The ability to sense our surroundings is so important that our standard equipment includes five paired sensory apparati: we have stereoptic sight, stereophonic hearing, we smell through two nostrils, touch with two hands, and can easily talk out of both sides of our mouth. To make sense of it all we use a bilateral brain and are often of two minds. Reaching a consensus with ourselves, much less anybody else, isn't just a noble goal, it's a flat-out miracle.

In the if-you-had-to-lose-a-sense game, touch for me had historically been the winner—or loser in this context. Smell and taste? Not my best, either. Fruity overtones and peppery-with-a-hint-of-regret were wasted on me; I bought wine if I liked the

label. But sight and sound? Had to have 'em. I wanted to be able to see and hear my grandchildren as they grew up. Okay, I could sometimes do without the hearing. It wasn't that good anyway. Neither was my eyesight, for that matter. It's not that I *couldn't* see; it's more what I would or wouldn't see. With this self-imposed limit on visual acuity, I may as well have done without sight after all.

That brought me back full circle to touch, which through the hands-on treatments I gave Diana became the sense that interested me most, but with which I could discern the least. My experience with touch was exactly the opposite of my habits with sight: whereas I expected to see what might not actually be there, I didn't expect to *feel* anything, whether it was there or not. But after a while, I did. Heat. Cold. Bumps and thumps. Pulsing and bubbling. And I had no clue how to correlate what I felt with whatever it might be. I suspect it was like someone unsighted from birth suddenly being able to see and having no idea of what to make of it.

I was encouraged, though. It was apparent that as with most new skills, I would get better with practice. Why in no time at all I could have a sense of touch that was as highly developed as any of my other senses, which meant it could be... would be... dismally mediocre at best.

So that was rather disheartening. I wondered why, after more than half a century, I wasn't more adept with my senses than I had been at five. It then occurred to me that my senses had actually been more acute at age five, and it was in fact the intervening decades that had dulled them. I suspected that more often than not I would short-circuit direct sensation and go straight to accessing a prior memory or association. I look at a Douglas fir and immediately dismiss it because what I see is just an earlier experience of one—which may have actually been a hemlock. When someone *always* reacts a certain way, is it really because he or she is "so predictable"

or is it because I am predictably and simultaneously recalling an earlier incident time and time again?

While Diana and I were trying to weave a healthy future together we had the misfortune of witnessing a marriage near and dear to us unravel. Over the course of two weeks I had a pivotal clash related to me by three different members of the disaffected family. Their stories were wildly divergent, barely hanging from the same fundamental framework, though each considered their version the incontestable truth. So what really happened? That's not just the wrong question, it's an absurd one. It presupposes there's only a single answer—and that it actually matters.

About this same time Diana and I had the unexpected pleasure of wandering through the grounds of a retreat in the Santa Cruz Mountains of California. We wound through the redwoods and salal, stopping at each in a series of benches inscribed with what turned out to be Buddhist precepts for training the mind. This was all new to me, yet somehow familiar. My first impression was that the precepts were very similar to the teachings of Jesus, just worded differently from a tradition hundreds of miles east and hundreds of years earlier. Each precept was a provocation; each more confounding than the last. Part of the inscription on the final bench read: "Undefiled by the stains of the superstitions of the eight worldly concerns, may I, by perceiving all phenomena as illusory, be released from the bondage of attachment."

All phenomena as illusory. That phrase has stuck with me. I think a typical notion of reality is not only illusory, but elusory and delusory as well. It's getting increasingly difficult—and less important—for me to know what's "real." I paint what I see. And I probably don't see it clearly. Or hear it clearly. Or take it in clearly through any other sensory mechanism. And then I screen those inaccuracies through a complex series of conscious and unconscious filters that

are likely even more inaccurate—not to mention inappropriate, historic, hysteric, and horrific. So what's "real" is hardly relevant compared to what I make of it.

"It's all in your mind" isn't the put-down that I always took it to be. It's simply a statement of fact. Whatever is in my mind depends completely on however I perceived it, however I interpreted it, and—this is likely the least stable variable in the equation—however I remembered it. That allows for millions of possible realities, so insisting I know what's real seems just a tad presumptuous. I now try to think in terms of "This is how I imaged it," which isn't too far from "This is how I *imagined* it."

Remember
to exhale

ear of public speaking is the Number One phobia in the
United States according to some surveys, probably conducted
by those who say they can cure it. It's ahead of death, spiders,
darkness, and heights, and is classified as a performance anxiety,
like erectile dysfunction but with the added trauma of a roomful
of witnesses.

That statistic was the first thing that popped into my head
when I was invited to give a 10-minute talk at a caregivers-only
workshop at Seattle Cancer Care. It also explains my knee-jerk
reaction when asked for a title for the talk, to which I squeaked:
"Remember to Exhale."

I'm not sure that it was exclusively a performance anxiety
issue for me. I was wondering more about whether I actually had
anything to say. It seemed presumptuous to offer advice to other
caregivers, especially when the workshop was geared primarily to
caring for brain cancer patients. We were done and gone with Diana's
metastatic lesions in the brain with a single swipe of the Gamma
Knife during the first week of treatment, so I assumed everyone in
the audience would be traveling a much more difficult road than
I had. But I also felt obliged to the woman asking, the coordinator of
the event and the fabulous nurse in the UW Radiology department
who was always so supportive and enthusiastic during Diana's
quarterly check-ups.

After a bit more thought, I decided that remembering to exhale was about the best advice I could give anyone, for anything. That didn't seem presumptuous. That was just common sense. Every martial art, healing regimen, aerobic exercise program, stress reduction guideline, and anger management course emphasizes the importance of breath: life-giving oxygen in; toxins and tension out. Can't get the good stuff in if I don't exhale, and it's impossible to relax if I'm holding my breath. I'd found that getting progressively worse news during each stage of the initial diagnosis and treatment made it as hard to exhale as standing chest deep in freezing water. It's hard to take anything in—physically, mentally, metaphorically—when there's no room in which to fit it.

So I figured I had my talk ready. Then I timed it. I needed to stretch out my message over another 9 minutes and 50 seconds. I added in the suggestion of cancelling all news subscriptions, as we'd done. Who needs more bad news? That was good for another five seconds. And that was it for the advice.

I ended up just telling a story, recounting the experiences that set us off on this… this… this Zen Road Trip, starting with Diana's idea of the Love-In. I hung the entire talk on the framework of the road trip metaphor. I mentioned the difficulty of deciding who gets on the bus when everyone ostensibly wants to help. The decisive factor for me was whether or not someone was indeed a caregiver. As soon as they morphed into a care-wanter, I'd kick 'em off. That only happened occasionally, and most of them made it back on board sooner or later.

Are we there yet? On a good road trip, that question is the quintessential faux pas. This was sometimes asked *of* us rather than *by* us, because the idea of an ultimate destination was somewhat meaningless. There was no there there in the sense of something up ahead that was identifiable or even desirable for us. The only "there"

for us was in the past, as in "We were there yesterday." So we were finding ourselves neither "here" nor "there" in terms of a position relative to anything else. There was no "You Are Here" arrow on our map, just a "You Are" arrow that didn't point anywhere in particular.

What "Are we there yet?" really meant was: Has she survived? Is she healed? Is she cured? And to answer those, I turned to the Online Merriam Webster Dictionary, which tells us that "survive" comes from the Latin roots meaning "to live above, over, on top of" and means "to remain alive or in existence; to continue to function or prosper." "Heal" is from the Old English "whole," with a first definition of "to make sound or whole; to restore to health." "Cure" is from the Medieval Latin cure of souls, with a first definition of "a spiritual charge." So, yes, on all counts. Diana has survived, she has healed, and she has been cured.

But will she still die? Of course. Of cancer? Who knows? That's certainly a possibility. Maybe even a likely possibility. But not the only one. Anything's possible… including getting hit by the very bus we were driving on this metaphorical road trip.

I closed the talk with a quote from Joseph Campbell that Diana had brought to my attention. "We must be willing to let go of the life we planned, so as to accept the life that is waiting for us." He didn't mean "accept" as in "be resigned to the life that is waiting for us," but as in accepting a cherished and unexpected gift. It's another way of saying, "remember to exhale."

I gave the talk to an audience that consisted of the organizer and her assistant, the guy and his daughter who spoke before me, and another guy and his wife who were to speak after. The rest of the workshop attendees were in a concurrent session about dealing with intransigent insurance companies. No matter. I still gave the mother of all exhales when it was over.

I still have the slides, though, in case you're interested…

Don't believe everything you think

The months after the blip showed up on Diana's CT scan were filled with exercises and expeditions into the extraordinary: explorations of any and all energy healing methods with hands on and minds off; extended forays into jungles of Buddhist thought and biblical allegory; excursions into the elsewhere seated under dolmens, walking around labyrinths, looking for chakra stones on the beaches of the San Juan Islands, and making bracelets out of glass beads and twelve miniature pewter goddesses. It felt like a crash course in slowing down time and wandering beyond the spectrum of visible light.

The blot was still visible on the scans six months later in December 2008, but there was no change in its size or appearance. We hadn't eliminated it, but we had apparently contained it. We just had to keep doing what we were doing, and for me one of the most valuable aspects of what we were doing had to do with *not* doing.

The hyperactive host and his animated dog on *Blue's Clues* encourage preschoolers to *stop, breathe, and think* when dealing with frustration. Smokey the Bear and Sparky the Fire Dog warn older kids to *stop, drop, and roll* when confronted by fire. And when embracing fate, the immortal lyrics of Rock 'n' Roll alert the rest

of us to *stop in the name of Love; Stop; Don't Stop;* and *Bus stop, bus go, she stays, love grows.* Everything important seems to start with a stop. Full stop.

It actually takes considerable effort to stop. It's not just a simple matter of inertia, because coming to a stop is actually the easy part. It's the staying stopped that's hard. If you follow the tracks of any Eastern train of thought long enough, you'll eventually arrive at the ghost town of Meditation, Nowhere—population either one or zero. All or nothing. Unity or emptiness. Presence or absence.

Why would anyone want to go there? I found the whole idea of meditation rather pointless. Just sit there and think about nothing? Why not just fall asleep? Which is what I did whenever I tried to meditate. Every time. For quite some time.

I discovered the trick to not falling asleep while meditating was… to keep my eyes open. I had a lock on the unfocused stare into the middle distance ever since Diana's diagnosis. It finally came in handy. I could now sit still, not fall asleep, and—as if to compensate for the uncharacteristic inactivity—watch my mind run off in all directions trying to round up every thought I'd ever had so it could parade them by for my reconsideration. And then I finally got it. The idea was not to try to think about nothing, but to get to the point where I have nothing more to think about. Nothingness isn't the goal; it's the starting point.

The bus stop at 3rd and Pine in downtown Seattle typically hosts a comprehensive cross-section of humanity: Brooks Brothers to Birkenstocks; confident to confused; intransigent to unhinged; medicated to probably-should-be. A dozen routes run along 3rd Avenue and most of the people waiting hope the person next to them is getting on a different bus. That stop provides an easy way to get out of Seattle and an even easier way for me to get into Nothing.

If you ever come across me in a full lotus position, please help

untangle me because it'll mean I'm stuck and likely in considerable pain. Meditative ambience is nice, but unnecessary because regardless of how I'm sitting or where I am, I imagine myself waiting at the bus stop at 3rd and Pine. My errant, misguided, and intrusive thoughts show up and wait with me, personified as passengers. One of the buses soon arrives, crowded with more of my unruly thoughts, and all those waiting climb aboard—except me. I'm joined by more who get on the next crowded bus, again leaving me behind. This continues until a bus finally arrives without anyone on it and no one's waiting at the stop but me. I ascend the three steps, take the first forward-facing seat on the right side, and ride to Nothing by myself.

There's obviously not much I can say about the place other than there are no services so I don't recommend going right after three cups of coffee. The important part for me was not in being there but in coming back, when the thoughts in my head that had been in full riot present themselves one at a time. Without the hubbub and clamor of their neighbors, it's easier to see that each one can be simultaneously inspired… and inane. Eternal… and ephemeral. Sacrosanct… and suspect.

My buddy Kurt once gave me a bumper sticker that read *Don't Believe Everything You Think*. I didn't think to be insulted until just now. At the time, I took "you" to mean everyone else, so I plastered it on the rear bumper instead of the steering wheel where it would've done more good.

My problem is that many of my thoughts reside in rent-controlled apartments in my mind and are understandably reluctant to leave. They are entirely unprofitable, and I'd like to evict them. I suppose I could renovate my mind in such a way that it is no longer hospitable to the long-term tenants—that would be despicable if I were a New York slumlord yet commendable if I were a Buddhist

monk—but you also never know what you're getting into with a renovation. Instead I decided to just open a methadone clinic in the lobby for whichever ideas needed rehab, which many did.

For instance—and since it was one of the first issues I faced in trying to meditate—my frustration with tinnitus had been particularly acute. I could never get to a place of absolute silence because after stripping everything else away—ambient noise, mental chatter, the organic rhythms of my lungs and heart—I was always left with the ringing in my ears. I bemoaned missing out on whatever was masked by this incessant hiss. After one of the earlier meditations, it occurred to me that maybe I wasn't missing any subtlety of sound; maybe I was just missing the point. Maybe the hiss isn't covering up something important, but is the important thing itself.

Arno Penzias and Robert Wilson at Bell Labs received a Nobel Prize for accidentally discovering the background cosmic radiation left over from the Big Bang. They were initially annoyed by the low-level noise that persisted throughout their experiments, but what they essentially took for tinnitus in their powerful radio telescope turned out to be the first hard evidence for an expanding universe. So maybe my hearing is exceptional, not compromised. Maybe what I hear is the residual peal of the bells that heralded the birth of the universe, the drone of the bees among the apple blossoms in the Garden of Eden, the sensuous and soothing voice of a New Testament God whispering into each ear: *"Shhhhhhhhhhhhhh. It's going to be okay. Shhhhhhhhhhhhhh, shhhhhhhhhhhh."*

Or maybe not, but at least I'm not bugged by it anymore.

To do…
or not to do

I t's hard to beat a Northwest sunset, especially when most of eastern Washington and good portions of Oregon and Idaho are ablaze. The particulate matter in the atmosphere from the smoke of a raging forest fire scatters light in a way that can be spectacular, sensuous, seductive.

We had some stunning sunsets throughout the opening months of 2009. The troposphere was contaminated with fallout from the ongoing detonation of the global economy and the dust kicked up by a marital dissolution nearby that continued to unfold with the slow-motion violence of a Peckinpah western. The little bubble of total focus that Diana and I had wrapped ourselves in for half a year was buffeted by storms and squalls of angst and anxiety.

In an effort to protect the air quality within the bubble, I started to spend more time outside of it. The challenge for me in addressing these external issues was how to engage without becoming entangled, how to remain detached from any particular outcome without becoming disinterested in the process, because, frankly, it would've been easier to not care.

I had learned enough about how energy flows around and through me to know to pay attention to the effects of that exchange rather than to the emotional pull of who-did-what-to-whom or why the world was going to collapse in financial ruin. I had also learned something about perspective: since I'd already had

the world collapse once, a second time is really not that big a deal. What I hadn't learned about was time. Every equation of production, progress, or profitability is dependent upon some limiting resource. Money. Material. Manpower. Or Time, the sand in the hourglass. Every minute outside the bubble was one less minute inside with Diana.

By April the tiny seed of a blot that had appeared on Diana's scan the summer before and had remained unchanged throughout autumn and winter had apparently germinated, and was on its way to full bloom. Why? That's a reasonable question for which there are only insensible answers. The most worthless of these—and the one I'll admit to entertaining briefly—had to do with my time outside the bubble and how I spent it.

Time isn't really a discrete entity. According to Einstein's Theory of Relativity time is inextricably wrapped up with space. Big deal. For that to matter to me, I'd have to be traveling at near-light speed. But the perception of time is surprisingly flexible even at the pace of normal life. It flies when I'm doing something I shouldn't, and it comes to a dead stop if Trigonometry is the period right after lunch. I can also make time, take time, and give time as if it were really up to me. So why isn't it? If I treat time as a limiting quantity it's not because it is, but because I let it be.

My Uncle Harmon had somewhere around a quarter of a million great-grandchildren. When Diana asked him how it was even remotely possible to have enough love to spread around to so many, he just smiled and replied: "They each bring their own love into the world." If that's how it works with love, then I suspect there's a way for each promise and problem and every delight and dilemma to also appear on the scene with its own measure of time. That's hard to imagine if I just see the sand slipping through the pinched waist of a three-minute timer. But when I think of

the endless sun-baked beaches and wind-blown dunes on seven continents and the suspended grains circulating the seven seas, the idea of time as a limited quantity becomes absurd.

Time only matters in the context of trying to accomplish something within (usually) self-imposed constraints. I can do one thing in a given amount of time, or I can do another thing, or maybe I can do several things concurrently or in sequence but I will eventually run up against a limit—not of time, but of doing. That's because time constricts with doing. That's the bad news. The good news is that time unfolds with being—and that's when it becomes an available resource, not a limiting one.

Diana's tumor started to grow again in 2009 because… because it did. We weren't particularly surprised by this development, and we weren't in a rush to do anything about it. First we had to sit with it. To be with it. To just be.

End of the world—reprise

There were several options available to us when Diana's tumor started growing again in April 2009. For the first time, surgery was on the table with curative intent. As attractive as that sounded, it made no sense to go through an invasive procedure with possibly debilitating life-long implications if there were still microscopic outposts of cancer elsewhere in her body. With metastatic cancer like Diana's, that is always a possibility for the patient and a near-certainty according to the oncologist. On the other hand, another round of minimally invasive targeted radiation would be far from definitive and certainly not curative. The Seattle Cancer Care tumor board could make no clear recommendation about treatment because there was nothing clear about Diana's extraordinary case: "Your guess is as good as ours."

Diana wasn't content to guess, and we also had a third option available to us that wasn't among the considerations of the tumor board: the return to full immersion in everything Eastern. Into her incomparable brain Diana plugged all the available data on her tumor, the assumptions and caveats about her condition, and the projections and probabilities of the treatments. Instead of a convoluted hypothesis, she posed a simple question to the trillions of cells that make up who she is: What do all of you want me to do? Then she descended into herself to dance with goddesses and mitochondria, to negotiate the interstitial spaces and allegorical

voids, and to consult and console the errant cells in the upper lobe of her left lung and the surrounding tissues that harbored them.

She did this several times over several days and finally got her answer. Surgery. That scared her. It scared me. But she was unequivocal about her intuition, and she trusted it completely. And that was fine by me because as it happens, my intuition was simply to trust hers.

This was not an easy surgery to contemplate. No one had ever removed a lobe of a lung that had been irradiated with such intensity. There was a long list of things that could go amiss. Uncontrollable bleeding from a brittle artery that might disintegrate under the scalpel was mentioned. So was death. Only a very slim chance of that, of course; probably about the same as Diana being alive three years after diagnosis. For me, that particular margin didn't carry the weight it used to. The surgery could be a beginning of days, or it could be the end of days.

Live each day as if it was your last. As if it were your last. Whatever. Whichever. Don't waste any of it worrying about grammar. That classic last-day sentiment is something I heard often throughout Diana's treatment. I almost certainly paid it lip service more than once, and likely passed it along, too—but alarms kept going off in my head every time I thought about it.

I think it was the frenetic urgency that made it unattractive. And the pressure! If I indeed had just the one day to live, or in this context, the one last day that Diana and I would be together, what would I do differently, really? That my mind automatically went to either 1) regret about what I might've done that requires amends, or 2) regret about what I haven't yet done (but want to) that might require amends, generated an artificial desperation in which I found myself with one foot firmly in an unlikeable past and the other in an unlikely future. I wouldn't want to spend my

last day like that. I wouldn't want to spend *any* day like that.

Diana and I had been more interested in making a day last than making a last day. The question for us was not so much about ticking off items on a bucket list, but rather how can we move a moment into the eternal, the realm where time has no meaning, where even meaning has no meaning.

By the time Diana's surgery rolled around, I had already discovered that I had neither the experience nor the imagination to adequately anticipate the marvels of this universe—or any parallel, intersecting, intertwining, or diverging universe, for that matter. I had historically shortchanged them all. I still do. So I try to be careful about what I wish for. I hate being limited by my own imagination.

When Diana was getting her initial chest x-ray in April 2006, I had hoped it wasn't pneumonia—that, to me at the time, would've been bad news. I got my wish. It was hopeless Stage IV Lung Cancer, instead. But I can't even say *that* result was bad news. We've loved the life we've been living since then. While each time the tumor grew would seem an obvious turn for the worse, some opportunity would simultaneously appear that would bring us closer to actually getting rid of it altogether. The prospect of the lobectomy surgery seemed to be good news. That the surgeon might be unable to complete it sounded like bad news. Neither was either.

Of all the books I've read in the past eight years, the one that has stuck with me the most was ostensibly written for children by Jon Muth. In *Zen Shorts* a giant panda named Stillwater relates a different tale to each of three children. Each of the tales is short, provocative, appealing, and likely appears in traditions other than Zen. In one, a Chinese farmer loses a horse. His neighbors offer condolences, "What bad luck!" to which the farmer replies, "Maybe." The horse returns the next day with a wild horse in tow. What good

luck! Maybe. The farmer's son tries to break the wild horse, but is thrown and breaks his leg. What bad luck! Maybe. The Chinese army sweeps into the village and conscripts all able-bodied young men, ignoring the farmer's son. What good luck! Maybe.

"Maybe" had never reached such heights for me. Its previously record was the top of the fence, the epitome of indecisiveness, procrastination, or dodge on its way to becoming an outright lie: "Can we go to Santa's Village someday, Dad?" "Uhhh, sure, maybe."

These days I'm a big believer in "maybe." The Chinese farmer wasn't avoiding a decision or withholding an opinion; he was simply acknowledging that he lacked the information to fill in the long view. I certainly don't have it. I'm not even convinced it's available. But openness to possibility is.

Diana's surgery was extremely difficult, prolonged, and ... successful. For the first time in three years, there was no visible cancer in her body. It is now five years later and there is still "no evidence of disease." Is she completely cured, or is it still possible there is microscopic cancer somewhere, somehow, sometime? Maybe.

Does it matter? Not really. If there's anything I've learned in the past eight years, it's that nothing is the end of the world. That's not exactly right. Nothing *has to be* the end of the world. If it seems like the end of the world, then I usually find I'm looking at it too narrowly. I've confined it. That's not the world ending; that's me ending the world.

Epilogue

Ancient rituals often include the passing of a sacred object—a shell, stone, sometimes a goat—that may or may not have any inherent magical properties but is imbued with them regardless simply by being part of the moment. The object is passed from one person to another conferring a transcendent quality, or removing one, or sometimes just marking when one participant stops speaking and the next one begins.

I had the great fortune to be engaged in such a ritual several months ago, in March 2014. Instead of a conch, a chunk of rose quartz, or an unfortunate ungulate, this rite of passage featured a deep red crystal, beautifully formed, like something you would find in Mammoth Caves. It was a whopping 2mm in diameter. That's $1/12^{th}$ of an inch, the space between the smallest lines on a typical ruler. I was appropriately positioned on my elbows and knees, forehead pressed to the floor, and—oddly enough—facing East. There was unintelligible moaning, which I was surprised to realize was coming from me and the kind of pain that—if it had to happen—I'm sorry to say I wished it had been to someone else. The stone in this case was being passed from my kidney to my bladder, though I didn't know that at the time. All I said was: *"Okay, body. You got my attention. What do I need to know?"*

As kidney stones go, 2mm isn't very impressive. What was impressive, though, was the other thing the emergency room CT scan showed: a mass at the south pole of my left kidney.

A month later—8 years after Diana's diagnosis and 5 years after her lobectomy—we've switched roles. She's in the waiting room and I'm in pre-op. I'm being poked and prodded and not unreasonably thinking about retributive justice. An eye for an eye… a tooth for a tooth… a needle for a needle…. This is familiar territory to just about anyone, mentioned in the Torah, the New Testament, the Qur'an, and much earlier, in the Code of Hammurabi. In all those references, though, it has nothing to do with exacting revenge, but everything to do with *promoting* justice… *limiting* retribution… encouraging *appropriate response.*

Whenever I'm laid up with a common ailment like the flu or a cold, the symptoms that make me miserable are not from the virus or bacteria directly, but usually from the barrage of white blood cells, antibodies, clotting agents, bodily fluids, inflammation, and fever that my body responds with in an effort to overwhelm and repel the invading force. It has always felt like overkill.

So there I sat, in the hospital smock that hid my nakedness just from me and no one else, legs dangling over the edge of the table, having turned not just the other but both cheeks to a cohort of pre-anesthesia residents. They were trying to thread an epidural feed between two of my thoracic vertebrae that had apparently closed ranks. Now that's an appropriate response to an invader, I thought to myself, a firm, localized, *you-can't-come-in-here* response.

As I was being repeatedly pricked in the back, I wondered if it were possible for the body to field an appropriate local response to the flu, to a cold, to any illness in a way that wouldn't be so taxing on the body as a whole. Not too much; not too little; a Goldilocks amount in just the right place. Then I wondered what I would do to help make that happen and immediately realized that was the wrong question. The right question was: *"What would Diana do?"*

That was easy. She would talk to herself, or rather to *"her cells."* She normally listens to them first and then engages them in conversation, usually through imagery, dreams, and meditations. I had neither the time nor patience for that. With all the jabbing and stabbing going on behind me, I was definitely in a telling mood:

Listen up cells, organs, skin, muscles… something drastic is coming your way. I know about this already. I approved it. You do not have to try to get my attention. What I'm looking for from you is an appropriate response, especially from you, capillaries and blood vessels. The surgeon says we'll need a transfusion of up to two units of blood. That's somebody else's blood. Not ours! That's just creepy. I don't want it. So blood cells, plasma, whatever else is in there… when your vessel gets severed—and lots of them will—don't pour out unless for some reason you have to. Just stop at the cut. Don't go shooting out like a fire hose or you'll get sucked up and thrown out. There's no future in that.

I figured that about covered it. The senior resident finally found the sweet spot at T7.5 and threaded the needle. They wheeled me into the operating room, put a mask over my face, and …

In what seemed like 1.25 seconds later, a very nice nurse in the post-op area was gently rubbing my shoulder, trying to wake me.

"… ughm gabla's yer name?" I asked.

"Tsomalie," she replied, with an indulgent smile.

"… umm asked you that before?" I deduced, mind clearing somewhat.

"This is the third time," she laughed. *"Do you also want me to tell you again how you didn't bleed very much? How you didn't need any of the two units of blood?"*

◉ ◉ ◉

Renal cell carcinoma of the clear-cell (conventional) type… Stage 1a… clear margins… If post-operative pathology reports were report

cards, that'd be an "A". It turns out that I may have had kidney cancer longer than Diana has had lung cancer, but while she has had to work hard to get into the 1% Club of 5-year survivability, I just have to lean back, relax, and stay out of the 5% Club of *non*-survivorship.

So what do I make of this bizarre turn of events? Not much, really. Diana and I do not live in the world of cancer; cancer lives in the world with us—with all of us. I don't think I know a single person who has not been touched by cancer in some way, sometimes tragically but more often, not. Over the course of our more than 20-year association with cancer, Diana and I have become inured to it. It has become familiar. It has become a circumstance—maybe even a condition—of life.

What it is not is the defining moment of a life, or at least it doesn't have to be. We have gained friends because of cancer, and because of it we have lost friends, even within the month. That is not the nature of the beast; it's the nature of life. But I have discovered that for me, when it comes to cancer—when it comes to almost anything, really—what I hope for, worry about, or am afraid of doesn't typically happen … but something better often does.

Acknowledgements

If there's a single message in what I've written it is that there is *always* another way to look at something. I keep reminding myself of that because my first take is so often wrong. That's the beauty of second chances. And third ... and fourth ... and ...

I would need all the chances I could get if I were to try to list by name everyone who contributed to Diana's—and my—healing. That would not only include our family, friends, traditional and integrative healthcare providers, co-workers at Lindsay Communications, the entire South Whidbey Island community, and essentially anyone we've come into contact with since April 26, 2006, but also many of their families, friends, and communities as well—people we've never met nor heard of... yet. Until I can thank each one of you in person, this blanket expression of gratitude will have to suffice.

Getting a story down on a paper is difficult, and in book form even more so. Many thanks go to the followers and commenters on my blog from which these entries originated; to our editor, Peter Guzzardi, not just for his keen insight and deft hand at easing the transition from the virtual world to the printed page, but for his huge heart and open arms; to Morgan Bondelid for her expert touch and artistry in the book design and layout; and our agent Anne Edelstein for her unfailing support and friendship.